# Last Artist Standing

# Last Artist Standing

## Living and Sustaining a Creative Life over 50

Edited by Sharon Louden

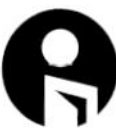

intellect Bristol, UK / Chicago, USA

To my dear

Aunt Kathleen,

for her love, courage, strength, curiosity,

and belief in me.

First published in the UK in 2025 by
Intellect, The Mill, Parnall Road, Fishponds, Bristol, BS16 3JG, UK

First published in the USA in 2025 by
Intellect, The University of Chicago Press, 1427 E. 60th Street,
Chicago, IL 60637, USA



A catalogue record for this book is available from the British Library.

Cover image: Jaq Chartier
*Blues w/8 Whites*
Acrylic, inks, dyes, stains & spray paint on wood panel
16"x16"
2020
Courtesy of the artist

Copy editor: Henry Johnson
Cover designer and typesetting: Holly Rose
Production manager: Sophia Munyengeterwa
Additional editing, copyediting, proofreading: Vinson Valega

Paperback ISBN 978-1-83595-097-5
ePDF ISBN 978-1-83595-099-9
ePub ISBN 978-1-83595-098-2
Part of the Living and Sustaining a Creative Life series
Print ISSN: 2516-3574 | Online ISSN: 2516-3582

Printed and bound by Short Run Press

# CONTENTS

# PREFACE

The common perception of artists today is often colored by romantic ideas of a mythological past where they would toil in obscurity hoping to be included in an exclusive art world one day and launched into fame and glamour. In reality, most are hardworking individuals driven by the need to express their truths, even if they are consistently undervalued and underpaid. At the same time, artists are more than just makers because they play significant, essential, and varied roles within our communities. Even if the majority do not earn a consistent income solely from their work to sustain a living throughout their entire lives, they contribute to the well-being of others and are pillars of free speech.

The 31 individuals in this book, all over the age of 50, show us realities of who artists are today. They share many different ways to sustain their creative lives beyond traditional gallery sales, which make up only one piece of the contemporary art ecosystem. Other tributaries of income include teaching, art handling, assisting other artists, starting art fairs, working in nonprofits, relying on the financial support of partners and spouses, etc. Because artists bring their creative thinking with them to *every* aspect of their lives, I argue that there is no such thing as a "day job." This outdated idea has no bearing on the real lives of the vast majority of them who leverage their creative capacity, energy, and skillsets to excel in everything they do. Regardless of whether they are making work in their studio, interacting and collaborating with others, or deciding to take another job for income, they remain artists. Every personal story in this book confirms how imaginative these contributors have been over the years in generating necessary methods to sustain their lives while constantly measuring and caring for their mental and physical health—ongoing concerns affecting every aging adult. These histories exemplify the resilience and dedication of artists who have consistently expressed themselves through their work over a lifetime. Their perseverance is relevant and inspiring to individuals in any field or walk of life, demonstrating the limitless possibilities of commitment and passion.

As an artist, I always thought I would never retire because I have always had a constant stream of ideas to fuel my creative practice. However, it is undeniable that our bodies break down over time. For many artists who are self-employed and live under a patchwork of funding sources, aging brings with it concerning unpredictability. Because of the inherent lack of value placed on the arts, security and retirement benefits are often unavailable to working artists, in contrast to those offered in the corporate or government sectors. Yet these mini memoirs inspire us with their common themes of solving problems to overcome hurdles faced over decades of worry, uncertainty, and lack of financial security, not to mention how each is devoutly committed to their work. No matter what is thrown at them, all 31 artists find ways to continue to express their creativity. Where the average person might give up, these remarkable individuals continue to share their artistic endeavors through choices in their lives and their work. They reinforce the notion that commitment leads to value in one's life.

For artists, what remains of physical work is equally as important as models of life experiences over decades that can be passed on to others in their journeys toward their own sustainability. I've compiled this anthology to amplify these lives as a resource not only for future generations of artists, but especially for those unfamiliar with the reality of what it takes to live as an artist.

Over the years conducting workshops and listening to thousands of creative people in hundreds of town-hall group conversations across the country and abroad, I have observed that there are two bookends of generations who do not usually interact with each other: artists younger than 30 and artists over 50 years of age. Sadly, as contemporary artists age, many tend to lose connectivity to the next generation as their visibility in the world shrinks. As certain contributors in this book highlight, though, intergenerationality leads to enhanced community building, which proves crucial to the productivity of artists and to our aging population in general. These stories emphasize that the potential for collaboration between generations is limitless across all sectors of the economy.

*Last Artist Standing* took five years to compile, through the pandemic, many hours of research, my up-and-down artistic life trying to continually sustain my own living, and delays due to my emotional responses to these essays. The foreword by Two Old Bitches (Idelisse Malavé and Joanne Sandler) confirms the adage that age is only a number. The conclusions written by Raheleh Filsoofi and Shervone Neckles, both working artists themselves, share their experiences of witnessing the lives of artists who continue to work in their later years despite lack of name recognition—a vital practice that keeps our histories alive. I also made a point to preserve the cadence and writing styles of each contributor as much as possible.

Over the course of those five years, we sadly lost three contributors: Valerie Maynard, Katinka Mann, and Audrey Flack. The essays they contributed to this book are among the last, if not the final, writings reflecting on their lives before their passing.

The main criteria when choosing who to include in this book centered on those artists who have been generous to other artists, continually creating community as their lives evolve. Generosity is important on so many levels, not just in our artist circles, but in every setting: generosity yields generosity, which creates more connection and opportunities for all of us.

These artists teach us that the meaning of success does not hinge on gaining accolades or prizes but is intrinsically connected to *longevity*, the gift of being able to express over a lifetime. It is not a coincidence that many who retire from a non-arts career turn to the arts to enhance their remaining years. The simple act of exercising that creative muscle—no matter what form it takes—brings satisfaction and well-being and extends lives.

If only people could see working artists not as a deficit to society, but rather as valuable specialists who have an array of talents and highly knowledgeable expert contributions, then the overall value of the arts would increase. Artists extend the lives of many while inspiring others to think more creatively. Artists in all disciplines are examples of abundance, because we have the ability to easily bounce back from failure, start something from nothing, assess and observe differently, and problem-solve like no others. To continue to think, discover, make work, and contribute to their communities throughout their 50s, 60s, 70s, 80s, and 90s, artists become beacons of great merit, inspiration, historical significance, and reverence. It is my hope that the pathways, skills, and tools revealed in these poignant essays will contribute to ongoing conversations that can only strengthen our understanding of how artists truly live. Their powerful journeys are footprints to follow so that our own voices can be seen and heard. ●

Sharon Louden

# FOREWORD

Now in our 70s, we are familiar with the real and exaggerated losses of growing old, as well as its frequently unsung gifts. In many conversations with other women in the second half of life, and some men, including more than 80 guests (so far) on our podcast, we explore how older women are disrupting expectations and restrictions born of gendered ageism.

Almost every last one of them confides feeling a stronger sense of agency than ever before with an irreverent independence from "shoulds" and "oughts." Feeling freer and more ourselves is our experience, too, and while exhilarating we know well that women who step beyond gendered margins to claim their power are vilified, and often called, "Bitch!" Some of us are taking that word back and redefining it as a badge of honor. For us, B.I.TC.H. is an acronym for Being In Total Charge of Herself, and in some cases, Himself. Putting "old" in front of "bitch"—as we did in naming our podcast *Two Old Bitches*—enhances its powerful transgressive spell, transforming proximity to death into a superpower.

The short portraits of artists in this book are illuminating and inspiring acts of solidarity and generosity that help others imagine how they can do it, too. In reflecting on similar stories we collect and share through our podcast, some recurring themes emerge. One that rises to the surface often is that, for many, making art is an irresistible calling that endures throughout our lives.

Our own artistic aspirations have deepened as we have aged. We both held demanding, full-time jobs in social justice organizations for most of our working lives. It was only in our 60s that we fully immersed ourselves in following our creative dreams and are thrilled at the way these are evolving in our 70s. Idelisse's love affair with clay over the past year has introduced her to an intergenerational community of teachers, students, and affiliated artists connected by craft and care, where age is no barrier with members making ceramics into their 90s. As a student at Brickhouse Ceramic Art Center, Idelisse saw and experienced the ways the community satisfies its members' every human need for a sense of belonging, mutual support, and celebration.

The importance and joys of a community of artists are not new to either of us. Seven or eight years ago we organized a small intergenerational group of women creatives and makers—writers, visual artists, musicians, and storytellers. Las Creativas, as we called ourselves, met every six or eight weeks to enjoy time to talk about our work and lives accompanied by good food, wine, and lots of laughter. We meet less often now and frequently on zoom (a practice we adopted during the pandemic lockdown). The bonds that connect us are still strong and enduring.

The podcast is another facet of our "art" in addition to writing, music, painting, and ceramics. Through each of these, we experience firsthand what it is to lose ourselves and our awareness of time when we engage deeply in creative practice. Not surprisingly, a raft of studies found that this practice helps older adults stay healthy and live longer. We can't help but imagine that the experience of timelessness is especially good for us when we are ever more aware of having less time as we grow older.

We are not who we were when we were young, and it affects the art we make and how we do it. And that's okay. Three dancers/choreographers we spoke with on *Two Old Bitches* reminded us that even when your art practice demands physical feats your body can no longer do, you learn to work with what you've got. Our art deepens and expands to encompass age's limitations along with the wide experience and wisdom we accumulate as we grow older.

This timely and resonant collection of essays offers a rich topography of diverse and multifaceted pathways that artists who have lived over half a century have taken to navigate and sustain their lives. Their reflections are a beacon for these times, demonstrating how the power of creativity, resistance, and community fuels the longevity of artists and the art they make. Our deep appreciation goes out to each contributor and editor Sharon Louden for standing up for art, for artists, for each other, and for the transformative power of their life stories.

Idelisse Malavé and Joanne Sandler,
*Two Old Bitches*

# AUDREY FLACK

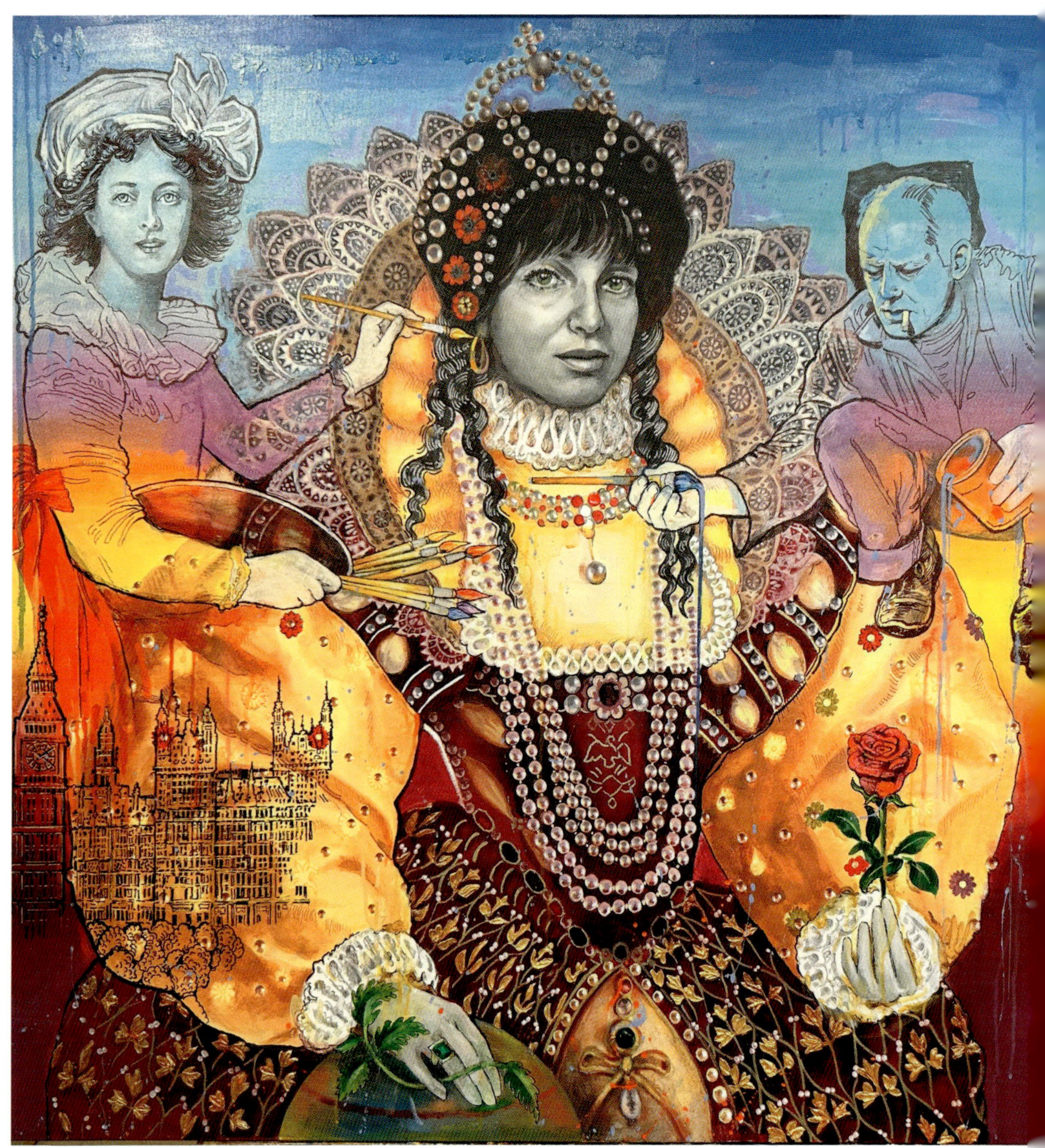

Audrey Flack
*A Brush with Destiny*
2024
40″x40″
Acrylic and colored stones on canvas
Courtesy of Hollis Taggart Gallery
Photography by Chloe Pitkoff

I HAD TO BE an artist. It was a physical imperative that started as early as kindergarten, before I knew what the word "artist" meant.

I was a hyperactive child, whose body and brain were sped up and in constant, irrepressible motion. I couldn't sit still, even for a minute. I slept little and arose hours before my family to draw, paint, scribble, weave scarves, string beads, and make bracelets, necklaces, and rings.

My behavior was not acceptable in the strict public school I attended, where children had to sit quietly with their hands clasped tightly on the desk before them. Even though I tried, I simply couldn't do it. I twisted and turned, wiggled and squiggled, and my legs vibrated up and down like a jackhammer. As a result, I was called "a very BAD girl." This label stuck with me until high school.

But in the first grade, a miracle occurred. The teacher gave us an assignment: an art project. "Make a diorama" she said, and that simple shoe box filled with paper cutouts changed my life. The act of making art calmed my brain, body, and soul. Suddenly, I could sit still, I could concentrate. Time stopped and extraneous noises and distractions faded into the background. Art does that, it stops time, and can cut through centuries.

Except for the diorama and one or two other art assignments, PS173 was an unbearable prison for me, a place where my spirit was broken on a daily basis. This lasted until junior high. PS115 was one of the most dangerous and decrepit schools in the city. But by that time, I was old enough to rebel and resist the imposed restrictions.

My parents were immigrants, and while they were both intelligent, they knew nothing about art or private schools, nor could they afford to pay for them. I had to rely on the public-school system and find resources for and by myself—and here is where I got lucky.

Through a friend in the building I heard about Music & Art High School. It was in an old gothic building situated high on a hill on 135th Street in Harlem. But most importantly, I could take the bus and it was free. I took the entrance test and was thrilled when I received notice that I got in. My spirits soared and life became beautiful. For the first time, I loved school. The next stroke of luck was learning about Cooper Union. At the time, it was the greatest art school in the country, and it was also free. I heard about Cooper Union's entrance exam late and had to scramble to make arrangements at the last minute. I took the grueling test and was accepted. I was on my way. This was topped off by being selected by Josef Albers to help him revolutionize the stodgy art school. Once again, I was thrilled to continue my education and to be going to the Yale School of Art. Although there are things I would have changed, like being able to study anatomy and figure drawing, I received a great art education and deeply appreciated it.

I was still a teenager when I completed my studies at Yale in 1952, and I returned to Washington Heights to live with my parents in their small apartment. I needed a job, and to start my own life. Jobs were hard to come by. I took almost anything I could get. There ensued a series of assorted jobs that covered the spectrum of being difficult, stupid, tedious, and disgusting.

I started as a Dictaphone operator in the Berlin & Jones Envelope factory, where I sat at a small metal desk in the center of a floor the size of a football field. The whole place shook from the vibrations of an enormous number of machines spitting out envelopes. My desk was placed right next to a machine whose mammoth jaws continuously opened and shut while applying sticky, repulsive, smelly, snotty glue to the envelope edges. The noise level was so great; you couldn't hear yourself talk. I sat at my tiny desk wearing heavily padded earphones (provided by the company) that didn't really block out the sound, but instead piped recordings of letters and business reports into my ears that I had to type out. These letters had been preciously dictated into a telephone by a company official, hence the name "Dictaphone." After six months of the madness surrounding me, I became so rattled, I quit, thinking "Dick-ta-phone up your ass."

After that, my job in a lamp manufacturing factory in Queens was a relief. It was better to be surrounded by people rather than the incessant overpowering roars of rumbling machines. My fellow workers didn't speak English. They were all Mexican immigrants, wiring lamps in the broken-down fire-trap of a building, while I was painting roses and Begonia blossoms on hurricane glass lampshades.

With my broken high school Spanish I managed to become friendly with my Mexican co-workers. During our short lunch breaks, I found out that they were being paid well below minimum wage. Outraged and upset for them, I reported this to the government labor bureau, who forced the employers to pay them fair wages. They were ecstatic and thankful; I felt good about it. However, the following week while everyone opened their envelopes containing their new and improved salaries, I opened mine to find a pink slip. My co-workers had an impromptu going-away party for me that day—a cupcake with a lit matchstick, and much gratitude.

When I got fired, or simply left a job, I would go on unemployment insurance—which was wonderful for artists. I could paint for up to 6 months at a time. This became the pattern of my life for the next few years.

I was an accountant's assistant for one week, adding up unending rows of numbers. This was a ridiculous episode since I am terrible at math and also didn't see the importance of the numbers matching and being exact. "So what if they were a few pennies off?" The poor old accountant became so increasingly enraged and frustrated with his unbalanced ledgers, that one day he had a stroke or heart attack and was carried away on a stretcher by a team of EMS responders. I felt terrible and never took a numbers job again.

My jobs got better after that. I worked in a small advertisement agency where I designed the "Royal Jell-O" box, and when Phil Pearlstein left his job as assistant designer to the famous European designer Ladislav Sutnar, he offered it to me, where I designed the logo for VERA scarves.

These jobs didn't pay very well and required my doing tight and restrictive art work, which was difficult for me being a free-wielding, paint-slinging, Abstract Expressionist.

The best of all was when I became a freelancer with the Jack Prince Textile Design studio in the heart of New York City's Garment District. I sat at a drafting table on the fifteenth floor of a factory building and created beautiful designs for blouses, dresses, draperies, table cloths, shirts, and ties. Our designs had to be beautiful or they didn't sell. The best part was we didn't have to sell our work; salesmen did it for us. They carried them around to top fashion designers like Christian Dior and Alexander McQueen, who incorporated our patterns into their clothing. We got paid per design, coloring, and repeat. Mine were the first designs to be printed on Terry Cloth, they became very popular and made enormous amounts of money for the textile companies, but the artists weren't unionized. We made a pittance, $64 per design, and $25 per coloring.

I designed paisleys and geometrics but became a specialist in flowers. Renaissance-style roses, Art Deco and Poire roses, peonies, pansies, and parrot tulips. Another great thing was that I wasn't physically and psychologically exhausted when I got home. I still had enough energy to paint. Other artists felt the same way—I sat between Paul Thek, Joseph Raphael, and Carolyn Brady; all serious working artists like me who needed to earn a living.

In 1958 I married a classical cellist and composer. By 1959 my first child arrived, and by 1961, I was the mother of two daughters, one of whom showed early signs of autism. We were poor, I had to sell my watercolors and paintings to help pay the rent.

I went on to teach at Pratt when Sidney Tillim—an artist and art critic—got sick and offered me his classes. I needed the money and grabbed at the opportunity, accepting every class that became available. I taught drawing, anatomy, two-

and three-dimensional design, and lettering. I studied and researched each subject before every class, sometimes staying up all night in preparation.

It took an hour and forty minutes to get from 104th Street & Broadway, where we lived, to the Pratt Institute in the outskirts of Brooklyn. The dean at New York University heard about my Pratt class and hired me to teach drawing and anatomy. I took subways back and forth from Pratt, in Brooklyn, to NYU, in Greenwich Village, and to the Upper West Side, stopping on the way home to shop for dinner. I cooked, fed, and bathed the children, read bedtime stories to them, and collapsed. When I revived, I got a couple of hours of painting in.

But I loved teaching and loved being able to develop the skills and talents of my young students. I am still closely connected to many of them.

After years of freelancing and playing in pick-up orchestras and string quartets, my husband got a steady job playing in the orchestra pit of Radio City Music Hall. Feature-length movies and spectacular stage shows featuring the famous Rockettes would alternate throughout the afternoon and evening. The orchestra had to be present for all shows, so my husband was rarely home. Aside from that, as it became more and more clear that our eldest daughter was severely autistic, my husband became less and less inclined to come home. This divide between us only grew and worsened—he became more and more demanding, irascible, and frightening; I was falling apart and had to get myself and my children out.

A year after our divorce, my life took a 180 degree turn for the better. My first boyfriend from childhood called, and within a year we were married. After a lifetime of trying to make ends meet, trauma, and stress, life became beautiful. Bob adopted my children and became a wonderful father to them, our marriage provided stability. I could finally breathe, sleep, and paint to the fullest of my abilities without painful and debilitating restrictions.

I went on to create some of my most powerful and meaningful work. The idea that artists have to live in poverty and despair is outdated and untrue. Most of us navigate our lives and achieve some sort of working balance to continue creating.

# BARRY UNDERWOOD

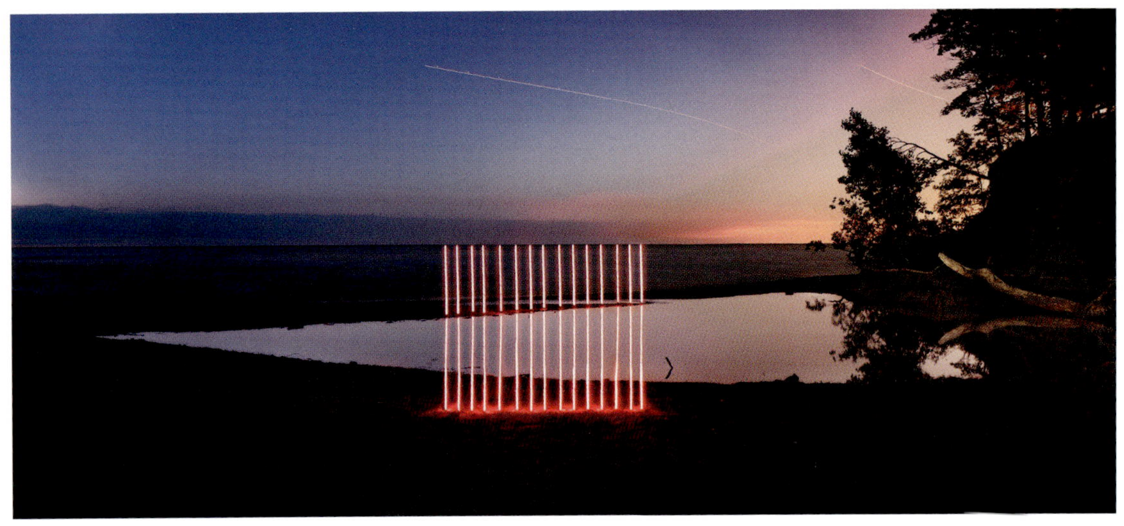

TEN YEARS ago I was diagnosed with Parkinson's disease, and yet, I think I am still in some sort of denial. This essay is the first time I have spoken publicly about the neurodegenerative disorder, how it impacts my creative practice and day-to-day life, and the myriad of ways in which I have been fighting back. It's a reckoning of sorts. A resounding admission of my reality. Here I am at 60—still trying to wrap my head around that too. I haven't fully processed what it is to be 50, to be 40. I am more invigorated than ever to make new work, but my body is constantly throwing hurdles my way. With Parkinson's, staying focused on a task is challenging, I cannot shift gears as easily as I could before, my dexterity has rapidly declined, and I face regular bouts of immobility. I am trying to figure out how to keep moving, how to adjust my studio to fit my needs, how to stay positive, how to not get depressed. I still need to get through the day and do something meaningful with my time in this world. I hope that by sharing my story, I can provide some insight into what it's like making art when you're not always physically and mentally capable of doing so, and maybe even empower someone in a similar predicament. It's nice to hear you're not alone in something.

Barry Underwood
*Huntington Beach*
2018
30″x70″
Pigment print
Courtesy of the artist

My creative career began a little later than average. My first lessons in art came while learning how to display fruits and vegetables while working in a grocery store in Boulder, Colorado, after high school. Through this simple task, I was shown the formal qualities of line, shape, form, and color within a produce display. The more beautiful the fruit looked, the more people would buy it. It wasn't until I was 22 that I decided I was ready for college. I enrolled at Indiana University Northwest (IUN) in Gary, Indiana, as a theater major because by the time I arrived for registration, there were only a few degree-related classes available that still had open seats. It was never my intention to major in theater, but as my education progressed, it would turn out to be quite impactful on my future creative endeavors.

In stagecraft class, students had three options for meeting class attendance: work on the set Monday through Thursday for a few hours a day, build sets all day on Friday, or crew the production. Since I was living with my parents again, I didn't have much of a social life. So, I selected all three options. The experience of building something creative, then watching the performers give their hearts to an audience nightly gave me an energy I never before knew existed. I built sets, crewed productions, performed in plays, and even studied ballet, tap, and jazz dance. I worked all day and late into the evening in the theater, only taking the occasional break to attend a class, after which, it was right back to the stage. I had found a home among creative people. In those theater days, we were kids in a playhouse. We learned to use our imaginations, trust our instincts, trust our creativity, listen to each other, move our bodies through space and be part of a family, a community.

During my junior year, I enrolled in a photography course. Slowly, photography was getting all my attention. I re-enrolled in the art department as a photography major, and made my way through a second BA in Art at IUN. Michelle Grabner was one of my professors and encouraged my artistic pursuits more than anyone else in the art department. This was at the very beginning of her teaching career, but she already had a knack for knowing exactly how to best support a young artist. Knowing she always had my back helped me further explore in the studio. Immediately following my time at IUN, I enrolled in the photography department at Cranbrook Academy of Art, studying under Carl Toth. He told me that my theater background is what set me apart in the applicant pool, and that he wanted to work with a student who would have a different approach to artmaking because of that experience. Carl was a generous educator. In studio visits, he would spend twenty minutes looking at your work and not say a word; he would be putting the pieces of the puzzle together. Then he would turn to you and just lay it all on the table, hitting the mark every time: what you were thinking in your approach to making, your influences and research, how you thought about art. He would always have a very deep and thoughtful conversation with you about your work, offering a direction on where to go, how to approach it, what to think about, and what book you needed to read. Carl was probably the person who knew more about photography than anyone and became a lifelong mentor.

In the summer of 1993, between my first and second years at Cranbrook, I worked as an assistant to a few artists as part of an innovative public art program curated by Mary Jane Jacob called "Sculpture Chicago: A Culture in Action". I was able to use my technical theater skills on different crews to facilitate and install projects for Suzanne Lacy, Daniel Joseph Martinez, and Iñigo Manglano-Ovalle. My encounter with Iñigo was brief, but it made a huge impact, particularly in my perception of the ways photography and video can be embedded in, and amplify, the voices of a community. Iñigo created a site-specific project in his Chicago West Town neighborhood called "Street-Level Youth Media (Tele-Vecindario)" that was focused on the community's predominantly low-income Mexican, Puerto Rican, Central and South American residents. Teenagers from the local high school used digital photography and made videos to correspond with one another about issues impacting their community. A massive block party was held, televisions were brought out to the street, plugged into power sources inside dozens of different homes and businesses, with each playing videos made for the project. Here my theater training came in handy as I helped run cables and install monitors and VHS players. Through this project, I observed the inventive ways ideas might be mediated through artwork as well as new methods for constructing a photographic image. None of the projects for Sculpture Chicago were executed through a single or traditional medium. Instead, installation, performance, site-specific projects, and audience participation were the focus. I saw new ways that my training in the theater, especially with the interdependence that medium requires, was relevant to artmaking. And most importantly, all of these artists were working with a community to make their work and enrich the place in which it was made.

When I was in college, I worked for a sculptor, Neil Goodman, who taught me that a studio practice is not a solo act. Like any organism, there needs to be a healthy, supportive ecosystem in order for an artist to grow and thrive. I recognized this communal approach from my own childhood experiences. My father was raised on a farm in northeast rural Arkansas in the 1940s and 1950s, where "pitch-in" and "help-out" were common language. Though he never said it outright, my dad taught me by example: to have a good work ethic and help others. Everyone in his community shared the load of every task, supported those who needed assistance, and taught the younger generation skills and responsibilities. These lessons are the foundation of how I base my current artistic practice.

My work stands at the intersection of staged photography, land art, and minimalist sculpture. I am interested in the cultural constructs of wilderness and the environmental issues related to human use and abuse of natural resources. I build temporary site-specific sculptures of light using electroluminescent wire or LEDs that are then installed in a landscape and photographed at night via a series of long exposures. Harkening back to my theater days, I see the landscape as a stage, and the light sculpture intrusions as the players. The team of studio assistants that help make all of this happen are the stage crew.

So much of what I do simply would not be possible without the help of others, and their contributions are paramount to my artistic practice. Well before the effects of aging and Parkinson's made studio assistants a requirement, I was regularly employing help in making my work because it's a physically demanding process. I need help carrying equipment, setting things up on site, preparing materials before a shoot, formulating a plan how to access and install in particular locations, and problem-solving in the moment. I have had assistants accompany me for location scouting so we can strategize as a team how to best utilize a site of interest. There's a lot of engineering behind each installation. We need to consider each aspect of a shoot beforehand to ensure everyone's safety and how to make the most of our resources and time together. The energy and support I get from having a small community contribute to the process are part of what propels me forward to keep creating new art. I love the collaborative process of making the installations with assistants who are my friends. We learn so much about each other in the hours it takes to plan, construct, and photograph a piece.

In 2011, my body's ability to keep up with my ambitions began to change. My left arm and leg started progressively, painfully, cramping up. At times walking became difficult. I had trouble with simple tasks such as putting my left arm in a coat and holding items. Typing was impossible. I was unable to move my fingers on my left hand. All of this was happening while I was the busiest I had been in years: I was teaching full time and serving as the chair of the photography department at the Cleveland Institute of Art, while also working on two ambitious commissions for the Cleveland Clinic and the Museum of Contemporary Art Cleveland. When I was in college, I endured a physical sensation where whenever I was stressed, my shoulders would get horribly tense. So at first, I just assumed my body was experiencing a similar reaction to being overworked and stressed. My friend, Joanne Cohen, was the curator for the Cleveland Clinic Art Collection, and someone I was frequently in contact with during this time. She was concerned about my ailments and knew this couldn't just be stress-related. As such, she made me see a sports physician, which then led to two-and-a-half years of medical testing. I saw neurologists, specialists, and physical therapists, while undergoing MRIs and other complex examinations that led to no diagnosis. In the midst of all this, I read Michael J. Fox's autobiography and was desperately hoping the same thing wasn't happening to me.

On January 9, 2014, my partner, Sarah Kabot, and I sat in a hospital waiting room in Cleveland, Ohio, staring at a poster of Michael J. Fox that read "Determined to Outfox Parkinson's. OPTIMISM - Pass it on." In the years leading up to that morning, there had been a variety of guesses as to my condition: a stroke, multiple sclerosis, pinched nerves, thoracic outlet syndrome, or other neurological disorders. Ultimately, it was a spinal surgeon who figured it out while he was examining me to determine if I needed surgery on my spinal column. But he didn't tell me then. He simply ordered a visit to the Movement Disorder Clinic. Before I was verbally diagnosed with early onset Parkinson's disease, that poster confirmed what I had feared. But I was also strangely comforted to have an actor who I had identified with in my youth be the one to break the news.

Parkinson's disease means that the neurons in my brain are gradually breaking down or dying, reducing dopamine production. I have difficulty walking, dyskinesia is a daily reality, I have lost a fair amount of finger dexterity, I often slur my words or speak too quickly, sometimes I get vertigo and become disoriented, and it can be difficult for my face to properly express emotions. Medications help me manage my symptoms, but I take several doses throughout the day and they have to be perfectly timed to be effective. As my medications start to wear off, my body becomes stiff, I have difficulty with small motor skills, and the physical act of "making" turns arduous. When I become immobile, my gait freezes; when I am stressed, I grow fearful and my decision-making turns more emotional than logical. I get aches on my ankles, knees, hips, wrists, elbows, and neck. Parkinson's can also mean a lack of motivation and depression, a closed-circuit reaction where each one amplifies the other.

The year I was diagnosed, I became very depressed and had difficulty making work. While it was good to finally know exactly what was happening to my body, and how to medically address it, I also understood the trajectory of how things were going to become more burdensome over time. My studio practice mostly took a backseat that year. Still, I tried my best to rise to the occasion when an opportunity to create was presented. Shortly after my diagnosis, I spent a month as an artist in residence at the MacDowell Colony. I connected with the playwrights that were in residence and felt a nice sense of community between our shared love of theater. I didn't make a whole lot of work during that residency, but I managed to create a few pieces that I am still proud of today. I see them as evidence of my ability to persevere amidst incredibly challenging circumstances. I am a maker at heart, and even in the darkest times, I will still find a way to create.

Cycling has been found to help suppress some of the symptoms of Parkinson's, so I began a regular riding routine. I signed up to participate in a program at the Cleveland Clinic to study the effects of continuous cycling on the progression of the disease. I raised money and rode for cancer research in the VeloSano Bike Ride, figuring that if I needed to be riding, I could help others in some small way in the process. This daily routine of cycling has proven to be a lifeline. In 2015, I was in Jackson, Wyoming, attending a residency at Teton Art Lab and still struggling with depression. I rode my bike a lot while in Wyoming and that helped my mental health and productivity in the studio immensely.

It took years to dig myself out of that depression. It wasn't until the summer of 2018, while an artist in residence at the Josef and Anni Albers Foundation, that I felt like I was really back in the game. I managed to overcome the feelings of despair and self-pity that had been plaguing me for years, and truly focus on making work. The studio space provided was fantastic, but it was the natural land on the property, access to the Albers archive, and learning about Anni and her work that really inspired me. I was more productive than ever. In two months, I produced the same number of complicated installations that would ordinarily take me a year to make. I created good daily routines and listened to my body's signals, finally learning how to work with, rather than against, my Parkinson's. And, it was just a big deal for me to get that residency in the first place. Until then, no one had recognized me for the use of color in my work. It was very affirming to finally be acknowledged for that aspect of my creative practice.

I know that in time, my Parkinson's will be more complicated to manage, especially daily mental wrestling match to motivate myself. For now, there is no cure for Parkinson's, but working on a project in my studio brings me joy and keeps me moving toward a goal. If I stick to my schedule for taking a pill, then I can get through the day with very little difficulty. However, that means I am extremely dependent upon my medication to keep me moving. Since each dose needs to be timed just right, I have to structure everything around the clock. I wake up early to take my pills, then go back to bed for an hour or so and wake up again once the medication has kicked in and I am able to move more easily and complete tasks. I have alarms set throughout the day not just for taking more medicine, but for tending to various responsibilities. I have to somewhat compartmentalize each day in order to function.

Fighting depression is a daily battle, but I try to create a positive environment for myself, aesthetically and socially. I try to engage in activities that will make me happier. I spend a lot of time in nature, whether that's going for a walk, working on a new piece, or simply enjoying breakfast outside in the sun. I bought a stationary bike that is more comfortable than my road bike so I can continue my cycling routine. The more I ride, the better I am. Music is imperative in keeping me moving as well. The beat gets me going, makes me feel proud, and gives me some swagger. If I don't stay active and motivated, then I get depressed. But with a good regimen and schedule, I can get through the day happier and with less symptoms.

Mentally, I feel young, but I am still frequently surprised by my body. The movements that I do and the way in which I speak affect how people interpret and interact with me. Anything from being sad for or frustrated with me to entirely misreading or understanding what I am trying to communicate. It has become a very big obstacle for me to overcome, and I can't help but take others' reactions personally. I have a habit of talking fast, and with Parkinson's, my words tend to come out rather jumbled and, at times, incoherent. So I am now in speech therapy, relearning how to use my diaphragm to speak while having greater awareness of my mouth, tongue, teeth, and throat. I love how it's connected to my collegiate theater days. I am learning how to bring back the voice that I had, and even giving Shakespearean soliloquies a go again, just for the fun of it.

It feels so good to feel young again! It's a joyous thing and I am feeling a lot more confident.

My partner, Sarah, has been the most significant force in my life. We share responsibilities in our home and support each other in our respective studio practices: technically, emotionally, intellectually, financially, and as each other's studio assistants. We met while we were each teaching at Interlochen Arts Camp in northern Michigan, a rich community of artists that we would return to every summer for over a decade of our lives together. In 2004, Sarah secured a shared studio space for us in an old storefront bakery in Cleveland's Little Italy. This is when both of our careers really started to take off. Having a studio outside of the home and workplace allowed each of us to begin building substantial bodies of work. We then also had a formal place to share our work with fellow artists and curators, ultimately leading to exhibitions. Undoubtedly, I would be lost without Sarah's endless encouragement and support. She's kept me motivated and energized when I've needed it most and has been a pillar in helping me navigate all this disease has brought our way. As my partner, the challenges I face with Parkinson's are just as much her burden as my own. I truly do not know how I would have gotten through all of this without her support. She's simply the best.

I still struggle every day, but when I spend time in my studio steeped in an idea, or am busy at school teaching and learning from the next generation of artists finding their voices, those are the good days. I've continued to participate in clinical research on Parkinson's while attending speech and physical therapy each week. Ironically, one of the photographs I made when I was first feeling the symptoms of Parkinson's is hung outside of where I attend my physical therapy sessions at the Cleveland Clinic. The Clinic has to think very carefully about what they put on their walls because of how it can affect patients and the friends and family that are there to support them. I'm honored to be included in the Clinic's collection and moved to hear that people have found solace and comfort in viewing my work while at the hospital. I've heard from cancer patients who appreciated being able to focus on my work while they were going through treatment, and a fellow person with Parkinson's who said one of my images reminded her of her backyard, thanking me for that familiar comfort found in a hospital. Most of all, I've loved hearing how babies seem to become fixated with my art. I can't help but wonder how their brains are processing what they're seeing. The Cleveland Clinic has helped me immensely throughout my journey with Parkinson's, so I'm grateful that I'm able to give back to them in some small way.

At this moment in my career and life, I reflect upon which achievements help to define success. Despite Parkinson's, I've been fortunate to live an incredibly fruitful life. My work has been shown in formal gallery settings, but it's also made its way into publications and online media spanning the gamut from *Slate* and the *Paris Review*, to Korean fashion magazines and the Weather Channel. It's hard for me to comprehend the myriad of spaces my images have ended up in. I've gained new perspectives and grown as an artist through residency experiences, my many years of teaching, and the rich community Sarah and I have built within Cleveland and beyond. I have had my share of rejections and my own meandering route, but I know I would not have any career without support from family, professors, colleagues, and friends. These encounters (some brief, some lasting), with artists, designers, craftspeople, writers, and musicians, have shaped the art I make, as well as my criteria for success as an artist. Since June 1996, I have been lucky to continue producing, thinking about, learning, teaching, or discussing art every day. Art surrounds my life, and I feel successful because of that fact. It is within this immersive context that I find new ways to be encouraged, and I can provide encouragement back to my community. This community of exchange is what keeps me going. And I try to stay positive as much as possible because negativity will take you out in a heartbeat. •

## COLLEEN COLEMAN

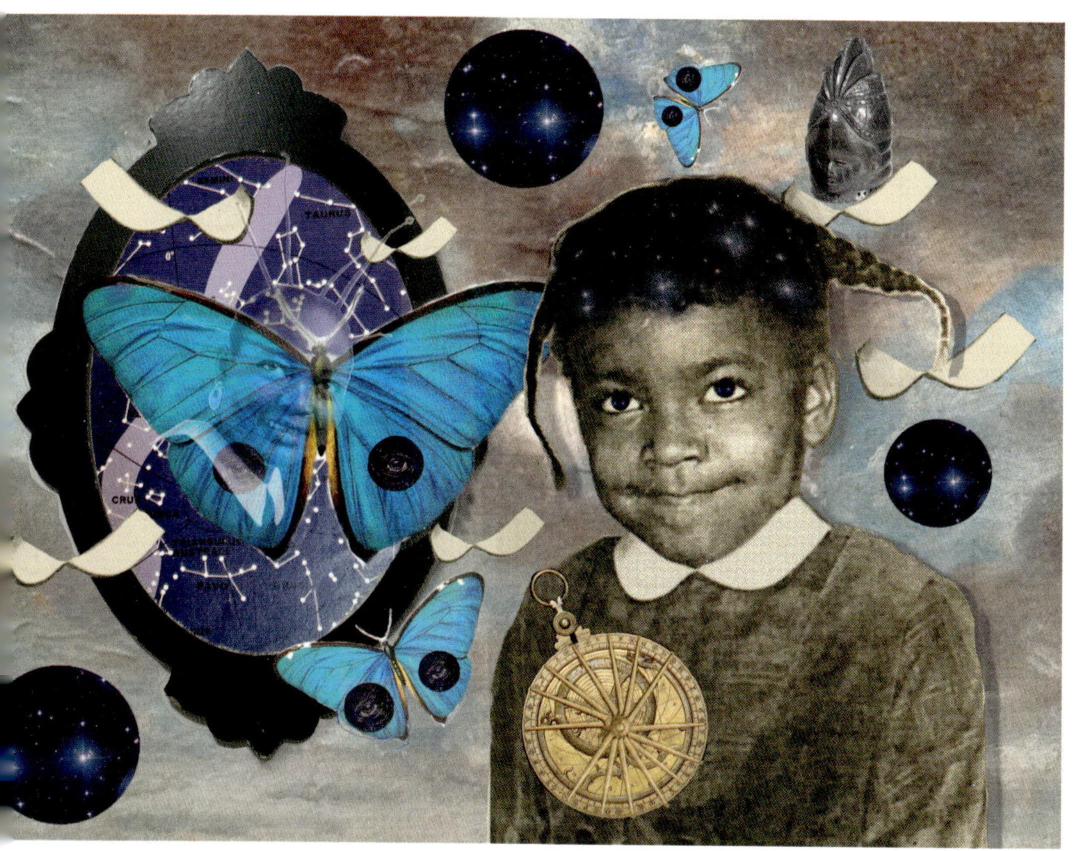

MY STORY IS one of a working-class family. My mother's work as a community organizer had a tremendous impact on my life. I marched in my first protest at the age of 8.

My maternal grandfather had emigrated from the Cape Verdean Islands off the coast of West Africa, an archipelago known for its people's ethos of hard work. My family story, like so many African Americans, spans the story of the African diaspora. My grandmother was part of the early years of the Great Migration and shared with me the magic of home cooking, the alchemy of food and love. In what would be my first cooking lesson, she showed me that with a few simple ingredients, and in only 45 minutes, one can provide a healthy meal for themselves from scratch.

My father and his family came north in the 1960s and 1970s. As a child, we would visit my father in New York, where he and other relatives had relocated from Darlington, South Carolina. Those childhood trips were the beginning of my love affair with New York City and laid the foundation for who I have become as an artist interested in history, class, and foodways. Education, hard work, service, and faith were my family's precepts.

I claimed my vocation as an artist by the age of 7, and there are many family stories that established the beginning of my creating even earlier. During my senior year of high school my family moved to a suburb located just outside of New Haven, Connecticut, where I was exposed to the Yale University Art

Colleen Coleman
*Awaken The Star Seed*
2023
36″x27″
Digital collage still
Courtesy of the artist

Gallery. The Yale campus and its art gallery became one of my favorite places to explore as a teenager. The architecture was designed by Louis Kahn. We would marvel at the collections of African and ancient art. We wandered through the galleries where we were introduced to and were sparked with creative possibilities by looking at the works of Albers, Twombly, and Martin Puryear.

I have always been something of an introvert and occupied myself with making art. I also met my first boyfriend who created comic books and played the bass guitar. His family helped to shape me. His mother was my third culinary teacher, his father a World War II veteran and jazz aficionado. His older sister introduced me to black writers and they became my second family. We were together for eleven years. They exposed me to the "Joy of Cooking," Ntozake Shange, Nikki Giovanni, Miles Davis, and Wayne Shorter. We would spend evenings after dinner listening to music on reel-to-reel tapes and talking about black history. Mrs. B would allow me into her kitchen and shared with me the secrets of making food that I considered to be refined and elegant black cooking.

I decided to attend Central Connecticut State University (Central) after high school and accepted into an Educational Opportunity Program (EOP). I am a first-generation college graduate in my family. I hadn't any idea what school rankings were and what the location of the school meant in the scheme of things. In 1977, at Central I met Michael Cipriano, my first painting professor. We shared a similar working-class background, but of course he, as a white man, made the leap from being the kid of a factory worker to a college professor; a very different route from mine. My exposure to painting solidified my path as an artist. I wanted to paint as color came alive for me and through it, painting became a visceral experience.

College had many hidden costs including housing, food, books, and supplies. I entered into a student co-op seeking a more practical career path. Student services placed me in a job at B.C. Porter Sons, the oldest furniture store in Connecticut. I studied manufacturing catalogs and did additional research on furniture history and design. I had found an area where my strengths could shine through, and I loved it. I saw interior design as a practical approach to a creative life; making sales, however, did not bring me joy. When I returned to school after my co-op experience, I decided to declare myself an art history major. I felt I needed to know more about the history of art to find a connection to the art world I so deeply wanted to be a part of. Unfortunately, I was only able to attend one more semester after losing my financial aid when Gerald Ford became president. Even with having a job, I wasn't able to afford to attend, so I left New Britain.

In 1983, I returned to Hamden, Connecticut, with no degree, nowhere to live, no job and an uncertain future. I began substitute teaching, which could be done with a minimal amount of college credits. While at college, I had befriended Michael Cipriano's son Michael, Jr., and we shared a passion for decorating and design history. He offered me a job working with him in New York. My lack of confidence caused me to skip the interview. That was the beginning of my thirteen-year venture into retail, where I worked in sales and display, eventually becoming a store manager for a women's clothing store. During the recession of 1990, I was laid off from my job and collected unemployment, giving me an opportunity to rethink my career trajectory.

I quickly sought advice from artists I had met several years earlier, including Barbara Harder, a printmaker and administrator at Creative Arts Workshop (CAW). She suggested I take classes, and I enrolled in my first painting class since leaving Central. It was 1990 and seven years had passed but I was committed to reconnecting with my artist self. CAW quickly became my second home, which was a place to explore my creative ideas and meet other artists. It was an amazing, energized environment. I was living with my musician boyfriend Paul Mills, who was the first creative person I knew who made a living from their art. I witnessed Paul's growth, going from playing locally, to touring internationally. Over our thirteen-year relationship, one of his biggest gigs was with Phyllis Hyman as her drummer and backup singer. I became aware of the possible ways to put together an income in nontraditional ways, taking on multiple gigs while doing the work I loved as an artist. Everything I did for work had a connection to art and my growth as an artist or sharing my creativity with the public.

A year after I started taking classes at CAW, Susan Smith, then director of CAW, invited me to teach in the children's department. Eventually I became the department head, and taught drawing to adults. My friendships with artists blossomed. I became close friends with Rita Haven, a painter I met in my painting class. She was like an older sister who supported my dream of making paintings that told my story. In that first or second year, I entered an art show sponsored by Artspace, New Haven, with the submission of a painted box. It was juried by the director of the New Museum in New York City. My work was selected for the exhibition and mentioned in a review with a photo of the piece in the *New Haven Register*, the local newspaper. Judy Burke, the only art critic in New Haven at that time, called the piece "a jewel." That experience was a signal to me that I had formed my life as an artist.

Paul and I broke up in 1997, and I was on my own, living a life of making and showing my work. I was actively volunteering on a gallery committee of Artspace, curating and hanging exhibits and learning all the skills that it took to run a gallery. The meetings with the gallery committee were my introduction to art theory and academic art attitudes. I spent a lot of time just listening and looking, making frequent trips to New York and the Studio Museum in Harlem, the Metropolitan Museum of Art, and SoHo when it was still the center of the art world. I began to sit in on Robert Farris Thompson's classes at Yale University. My fellow committee members treated me with respect and regard, but I felt like an imposter. It was sometimes painful as I was not formally educated in art, yet surrounded by fellow committee members who had attended Carnegie Mellon and Yale, who were teaching at colleges in the surrounding area and exhibiting nationally and in New York.

By 1995 I had fashioned a life that gave me the flexibility to make art and survive as an independent adult working as many as five jobs at a time, teaching art as a visiting artist for the

New Haven Board of Education, preparing kids in New Haven schools to visit the Yale Art Gallery, and conducting residencies at area schools through City Spirit Artists. Over the years, I have participated in artist-in-residences, worked with community organizations, the Yale Art Gallery, New Haven Jail, the New Haven Police Academy, and the Kingswood Oxford School.

In the early 1990s, established arts institutions feared decline, sought to create new audiences, and understood the necessity of diversity. The National Endowment of the Arts (NEA) began reducing funding for individual artists while investing more in community arts. In 1994, the Urban Artist Initiative (UAI) came to New Haven, offering professional development for artists. UAI changed my life. I participated in weekly workshops and was given an artist/mentor in Suzan Shutan. Meeting Suzan was like running into a storm. She was energetic and tenacious and encouraged me to get out of my own way. That same year, I became the program coordinator for UAI as the program expanded to a new city and I put myself forward to take on the task of helping to launch the newest site. We established sites in 10 cities around the state of Connecticut and changed the cultural landscape. The cultural diversity of the program had never before been seen in Connecticut. Many ethnic communities, including Haitian, Tibetan, Greek, Indian, African-American, Chinese, Puerto Rican, Cape Verdean, Polish Russian, Ecuadorian, Brazilian, Colombian, and Cambodian, felt the impact by the participants who were performers and makers.

Maryland Grier, the director of UAI, hired me as program coordinator and later entrusted me with the job of curator of visual arts exhibitions. She trusted my arts acumen and critical eye, and her boss Jean Schensul, the director of the Institute for Community Research (ICR), supported my art practice with a flexible schedule and encouraged my practice.

It was also one of the most productive times of my arts career. I had a studio at the Erector Square building in New Haven. Even with all the work at my day job, invitations to join various boards and review committees, I managed to make my own work. I became a board member for Projects for A New Millennium, Inc., founded by Joy Wulke. Joy and I became friends, and she was a mentor. She told me success is not about being the greatest artist, it's about continuing to make the work. The artist keeps working. Don't ever stop making.

I had the energy and drive to have my studio practice and exhibit work. I firmly believed New Haven was the arts capital of Connecticut. Recognition for my work as an artist came locally and regionally. My first museum exhibition was curated by Dr. Frank Mitchell, curator and historian of the Amistad Center for Arts and Culture at the Wadsworth Atheneum. In 2000, with the new millennium, I was invited to my first show outside of Connecticut after a residency at Vermont Studio Center. I exhibited work in a group show at the Utah Museum of Contemporary Art, in Salt Lake City. Museums and community gallery invitations were plentiful but there was no offer of gallery representation and frankly few private sales of work.

As the times and the government changed to the Bush administration, so did funding for the arts overall, including grants from the NEA which dried up. The Connecticut Commission on the Arts also decided to move its focus away from funding individual artists. Feeling the need to be credentialed, I decided to return to school in 2004 and completed my undergraduate degree in June 2007. I took on a new role at the Institute for Community Research as artistic director. We continued to provide exhibition opportunities in the gallery to UAI artists and the larger community. The commute to Cambridge College in Springfield, Massachusetts, from New Haven was a bit more challenging and with homework, my art practice suffered. I could no longer afford my studio. I moved in with my family to focus on school.

The amazing thing is, in 2005, I was included in an artist project by Professor Imna Arroyo, from Eastern Connecticut State University, who created a video and curriculum for schools introducing the public to five women artists of color. Voyages of Time and Place was the curriculum that included myself and four other artists, as we toured the state with several exhibitions. The final stop was an exhibition at the Benton Museum at the University of Connecticut (UCONN) in Storrs. The director, Sal Scalora, purchased not one, but two works from me for the museum's permanent collection. That year I also received a Connecticut Commission on the Arts Fellowship for Painting.

In 2008, ICR lost its funding and I would be losing my job. Not fully secure in any of the positions I had held, I decided to take a risk on myself and looked into MFA programs. I didn't have a BFA but a Liberal Arts degree and I had only attended public schools. No one in my family was in higher education or was a professional. Making art has always been central to my life's goals. I applied to the MFA program at the School of the Art Institute of Chicago (SAIC) and was accepted into their sculpture department. I moved to Chicago in 2009. Living in Chicago was a difficult and challenging experience for me. I found my space mysticism in the likes of Sun Ra, which has historically been a part of Chicago history and the city's energy. Perhaps it's due to the city's placement on the edge of the lake. It's an Axis Mundi. SAIC's history in itself, and specifically that of Louis Sullivan, fascinated me, and I often found myself visiting Roseland Cemetery. Reflecting back on it, I found solace with a professor emeritus named Preston Jackson, who encouraged my coming to the school. I volunteered at the renowned South Side Community Arts Center and was the graduate assistant to Faheem Majeed and Drea Howenstein. In my class, there was only one other classmate over 35. How was it people with such little life experience were working on what would become the central themes of their life's work? There was a lot of talk about ending the terminal degree of MFA and extending it to a PhD program. It all converged to make for two years of hurdles and challenges. Championing me every day from afar were my mother and older sister Laurel. I graduated the day after my 50th birthday in May 2011. I came away with more knowledge of art worlds and how they worked and with a different sense of the academy. I had achieved my goal: an MFA from one of the most historically significant art schools in the world. After graduation, I decided to return to the East Coast as my mother's health was failing and I needed to be close to my family.

In 2011, I moved to Brooklyn, New York, and found a place I could afford with a roommate in Bushwick. I paid my rent with the earnings from my part time work at the Museum of African Diaspora (MoCADA), an artist-in-residence at Weeksville Heritage Center, and the studio in a school in New

York City, but the total income from all of my jobs still wasn't enough. I couldn't afford to live in New York with just part-time jobs, and I wanted stability, art materials and health insurance. I also wanted to be of help to my family. I had to commit to finding a full time job and teaching children was a natural area to explore. In 2011 there were hiring freezes at state colleges and universities and the economy still hadn't recovered from the financial and housing crisis. I spent days visualizing how life would be with a job, a space of my own, food in the fridge and time and space to create art. One afternoon, at 47th and 5th Avenue at Rockefeller Center, I ran into Nabia Meghelli, who is the daughter of Algerian-American artist Fethi Meghelli and educator Barbara Greenwood. Nabia's parents and I were karmically connected since I was 16 years old. They mentored me, hired me for some of my first artist residencies, and saw me off to Chicago when I left Connecticut. Fethi worked with my mother and had spoken to me about my college plans when I was 16. Years later, we both worked at CAW and would exhibit together. Meanwhile, Barbara was a teacher/principal at the High School in the Community, an alternative high school in New Haven based on the Hyde School academic model. In 1992, Barbara hired me to teach one of my first artist residencies in New Haven.

Nabia's parents were integral in my life. She told me the school she was working for was looking for an art teacher. The school was a charter school in Harlem. I am still teaching art at that same elementary school nine years later; I'm 63 years old. The community has seen me through the losses of loved ones, the last being my mother in 2020, but also the re-emergence of my art practice.

Three years after my mother's death, I have once again re-committed myself to my art practice, something my mother encouraged throughout my life. I am heeding her advice—"Colleen do your work, it's important"—and the universe is working for my good. 2021 began with an invitation to re-perform a performance installation piece at Eastern Connecticut State University. The school purchased the drawing for their permanent collection at the fine arts building. It was like stepping into myself and my purpose as I prepared by writing and researching every molecule, moment, and breath: I felt awakened. The performance was entitled *Drawing Performance: 4th Iteration Wake.* The piece was a celebration and memorial to my ancestors known and unknown. My women's healing circle held me that day and so many loved ones wished me well from around the country. As I completed my first durational performance in 10 years, I drew nonstop for two and a half hours. That action opened me up. In the following weeks, I began applying for opportunities for residencies and was blessed to have a new confidence in my purpose.

I am fulfilling my dreams and doing what I love, connecting with people of all ages, telling the stories of my ancestors and making space for those like me who come after me. I don't have any birth children but I have thousands of children. My life has been one of sharing, and making my art. Things I love. It is not solely for myself but it is a recognition of what was poured into me. My students inspire me to continue exploring to push forward in the unearthing of our history. I believe in Sankofa to learn from the past, to build a future, and I encourage them to go beyond themselves, their neighborhood, and the life and circumstances they were born into. They must have hope to continue in one of the most complicated and inspiring places in the world.

I have achieved my goal of being a lifelong learner of history, culture, philosophy, and the heritage and tradition that shape us. Don't underestimate the insights of children, especially those who have already experienced extreme conditions of living. These kids love art and some have, like me, proclaimed themselves as artists at their very young age, sharing with me their love of art.

I know I have done something right. It used to frighten me when children would tell me they wanted to be an artist like me, not wanting them to know what a struggle it has been. Now I realize I am preparing an army of artists who will be creatives who are open to their creative expression. They will speak loudly and boldly, and yes, at 5, 6, 7, 8, 9, and 10 years of age. They proudly declare themselves ARTISTS.

2022 was a very good year for me as it was a push in the right direction. A residency at Chautauqua School of Art helped me to see my dream can be a reality. To connect with a community of artists from such a diversity of backgrounds was like a homecoming.

I've retired from teaching full time and now fully committed to my practice. I am busy applying for residencies and opportunities and discovering what it means to be my authentic self every day. Exploring, asking what this human experience is about, learning what stories need to come through me with the hopes of adding something of value to the world, is of importance. Service is still central in my thinking and the love of my people and all of humanity's survival. But now I have, and recognize, the freedom to prioritize my work and the stability that retirement offers. It is time to focus my energy on my studio practice. The idea of not seeing the children and their families is difficult to imagine, but it's time. ●

EVA LUNDSAGER

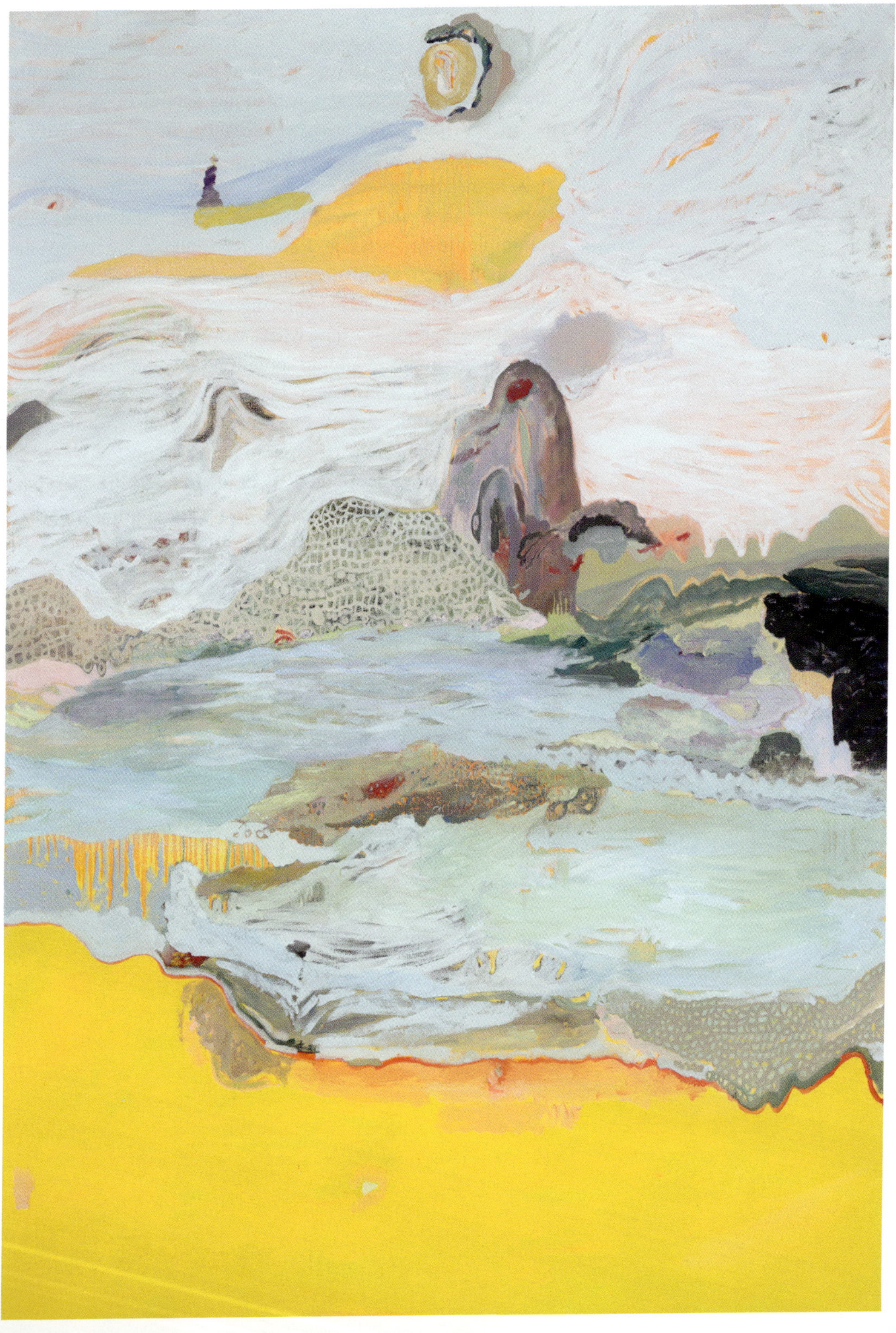

Eva Lundsager
*A pause*
2021
74″x64″
Oil on canvas
Courtesy of the artist
Photography by Julia Featheringill

I GREW UP in Maryland, about 20 miles north of Washington, DC, in a small town called Ashton. I went to the local public school and was friends with kids who showed their cows at the county fair and I took sewing lessons with the local 4-H club. My parents had moved to the United States from Denmark in 1952. My father had an engineering degree, but there weren't many jobs in Denmark in the years immediately following World War II. So, with two small children, my oldest brother and sister, they moved to the United States when the Dupont company offered him a job. Mom and dad had two more children here, my other sister, and me. I'm the baby, born in 1960.

My brother-in-law, Stephen, recently said that he's always thought of my mom as an artist, which took me by surprise. I hadn't thought of my mom as an artist, and I don't think she did either, but she's always made things, clothing and curtains, embroidery, knitting, weaving, and braided rugs. One time she entered a sweater she made in a fibers exhibition, and was told by the juror that she would have won first prize except the juror suspected she had made the sweater on a knitting machine—that's how good it was—and, no, it wasn't made on a machine. My dad, too, was always making things. He loved working with wood, and he made toys, imaginary creatures, and bowls; built our bunkbeds and bookshelves; crafted exquisite cut-paper valentines for us; and painted a few pictures too. My sister and I were always making things, drawing, sewing outfits for our trolls, and doing whatever crafts were on-trend in the 1960s and 1970s (remember Creepy Crawlers made with goop? Wire flowers dipped in plastic? and many macramé plant hangers). Our family regularly visited the Smithsonian museums, which are free, and if admission had been $20, we probably wouldn't have gone so often. Why aren't all museums free?

I was never much for school, and I graduated from high school when I was 16, in 1977. School felt like a distraction from my work, which was making things. My saving grace in high school was my art teacher, Mrs. Ruyter, now Lynn Schulte LaValley, and she would drive me to a ceramics program affiliated with Antioch College, called the Visual Art Center. Lynn was getting her masters in a fine art degree in ceramics, and I was taking wheel throwing classes with her, alongside adults working toward their degree. The year after I left high school I spent every weekday there, working part-time in the store and continuing to take classes. By the time I was 17 I had done the equivalent of a master's degree in ceramics. It was there, at the Visual Art Center, that I learned how to work hard at my art, as artists do, every day. It was the first time I felt at home in a school environment; it was school but it was different, I was doing work I cared about, in a community of artists and art students. The other students were all much older than me, and after a year or so, in the spring of 1978, I realized I had to grow and move on, and get out of my parent's house. I enrolled at the University of Maryland that fall, just before my 18th birthday. I can remember half-heartedly filling out the application, not really wanting to go to college, but not knowing what else to do. I didn't try too hard, I knew I would get accepted, as it was much easier to get into than it is now. Both my sisters were already at the University of Maryland, and my brother had graduated from there a decade earlier. Hanne is two years older than me and she was really my go-to friend those first years of college. Meg was teaching economics and working on her graduate degrees, and she helped me sign up for classes and looked out for her younger sisters. I still didn't like school, but their presence helped me a lot.

It's hard to pinpoint why I disliked school so much, a feeling that continued through my first couple of years of college before

I committed to painting. I felt trapped when I was in a classroom. Looking back, it was really hard for me to talk to people; it's like I was walking around inside out. I was shy, but I knew I liked art, and I dreamed of a life spent making things. Or maybe I was just bored. Studying ceramics at the Visual Art Center when I was a teenager was the first time I liked being in school. It seemed like you had to be a freak or a jock, and I was someone who wanted to make things and look at things and think about things other people had made, and I didn't like being in large groups.

Our parents always encouraged us to find work we enjoyed, and as I became more and more interested in art, Dad suggested I look into working at a museum, organizing shows. Neither of us knew the word curator, and I knew I didn't want to work with artists, I wanted to be an artist. Still, I was afraid I wouldn't be able to support myself. I was afraid I'd be a burden, or a disappointment to my family, so I spent my first three years at the University of Maryland in College Park without a major, mostly taking studio art classes, but also taking other classes, trying to find a more practical profession, though I'm not sure how practical anthropology is, and I just daydreamed my way through an economics class. In early 1981 I got mono and dropped out of college. When I was better I drove across country with my friend Holly, who was moving to San Francisco, and I tagged along for the adventure. I decided to stay there, and I supported myself with temp jobs, including a stint as receptionist for then State Senator Milton Marks, where my chief duty was writing sympathy letters to constituents. My evenings were spent hanging out with Holly and new friends. People were just starting to talk about a gay cancer, but at that moment it felt like it would quickly blow over. I didn't take it too seriously until a year or so later when more people started dying. Few of our gay, male friends from those days survived.

After six months in San Francisco I grew pretty bored with my jobs, and while San Francisco is a great city with lots of fun to be had, I didn't want to make a career of living there. I decided to finish college and finally commit to what I really wanted to do, the thing I loved and felt part of like nothing else, making art. So in January 1982, I returned to the University of Maryland and threw myself into painting. I stopped trying to force myself into a more practical profession and finally, started to like school. And I started to think of myself as an artist.

What brought me back to painting? I think it's more that ceramics was a detour. The 1960s had a lot of people crafting, and painting seemed like something just for the rich, and I wasn't rich, and pottery seemed like something more accessible, something anyone could own, whereas painting seemed more elitist. So I took a little detour. Recently we brought out some of my ceramics, and it's fun having them around, like paying homage to younger me, and they're better than I remembered.

The University of Maryland in the 1980s was amazing. My teachers included artists David Driskell, Sam Gilliam, Nick Krushenick, Anne Truitt, Claudia DeMonte, art historian Josephine Withers, and critic and theorist Jack Burnham. They all lived their commitment to art. It's so hard to put into words, but they were serious about their art, a seriousness I recognized, that felt familiar, that felt like home. Art was central to their being and didn't have to be justified. Mrs. Truitt, as we called her, gave a talk in class one day on what to expect when a museum is giving you a retrospective, giving each of us the gift of imagining a future where our work was valued and honored. Sam Gilliam would meet us at galleries in Washington, DC; he always treated us with kindness and respect and laughed easily, making class feel like community. I am so proud to have learned from these artists, to visualize my own life as an artist. How lucky I was to have been there, working with these great artists, and when tuition was only around $400 a semester.

Lucky too that college is where I met my husband, Paul, who was making incredible art even as he was announcing to everyone that once he graduated he would never make art again, a promise he's pretty much kept. In the early 1980s Paul was playing in Washington, DC, punk bands and volunteering at the Washington Project for the Arts. We would see all the shows in DC, music and art, and regularly drive to New York to see more art. Paul had come to the United States from Korea when he was 9. Our Danish and Korean families actually have a fair amount in common: our parents all lived under foreign occupation, with experiences that stayed with them throughout their lives.

My dad spent nine months in a Nazi prison at age 19, when he was caught working with the resistance, and Paul's mom and her family had to flee Seoul when North Korea invaded. His uncle was captured by the North and never seen again. And while both our parents believed in working hard, they also valued the beauty to be found in the world, in music, art, and nature. And even though they had difficulty understanding each other, our mothers became friends.

After I graduated from the University of Maryland in 1984, my teacher Claudia DeMonte encouraged me to go to graduate school and she helped me figure out where to apply. I spent the year between undergrad and graduate school working temp office jobs to save up a little money, and I paid for a course in "word processing," as they called it then, so I would have a skill that paid a bit more than just answering phones. I got into every school I applied to, but chose Hunter College, as it was the cheapest, in New York City where the art world was, and not too far from Paul, who was still in college in Maryland. Hunter College's classes were held mostly in the evening, so I was able to work temp jobs during the day, just enough to pay my bills.

A few months after moving to New York in August 1985, Claudia set up an interview for me with her gallery, the Gracie Mansion Gallery, and suddenly I was a registrar. The Gracie Mansion Gallery was one of the best-known galleries at that time, and I could not believe that I was allowed to touch the art; it felt so precious, and I was honored to be there. The first show after I began was a solo exhibition of Peter Hujar's work. I still remember typing up the price list, where his iconic photos were $350. I was definitely not the ideal "gallerina," as I was super shy and kind of awkward, but I did a good job with the paperwork and keeping track of the art.

Before I moved to New York, I had imagined that any artist whose work appeared in an art magazine must be a millionaire. Soon I learned that most of the artists were working in their apartments or in cramped studios, and doing whatever they could to give themselves maximum studio time. This was not discouraging; it was inspiring, and helped me imagine how I could make a life for myself as an artist. I learned so much.

I'm still friends with Gracie and her partner in the gallery, Sur Rodney (Sur), and some of the artists from the gallery, too. Like my undergraduate teachers, they gave me a vision for how I could make a life, and I was just so happy to be part of their world, which was now my world, too. Many of them came to the opening of my MFA thesis show in 1988, my first solo in New York, and I still have the guest book signed by the artists, some of them now long gone.

One day I was seeing a show on the Upper East Side of New York City, I overheard people behind the desk talk about looking for an art handler. I told Paul, he called the gallery, and found himself with a job before he even moved to New York. After taking his last final exam, he got on a train, didn't attend his own graduation, and started his job the next day. I thought Paul would find new bands to join and we would live together as young artists in New York. I suppose we did that, but Paul soon became more and more interested in working with artists. He volunteered at White Columns, then on Spring Street, did tons of studio visits, and soon enough started moving up in alternative art spaces, and later, museums. Together we were hanging out with our artist friends, such as Judy Glantzman, Maya Lin, and Gail Fitzgerald, seeing all the shows and going to openings. I was trading studio visits and art, our living room was my studio, while I supported myself with temp jobs. I had the world's worst health insurance and didn't go to the dentist. And then friends started getting shows. Our friend Carl Ostendarp was in a show at a new gallery, Stephanie Theodore, and he told Stephanie about my work. Stephanie visited my studio and soon offered me a show. At the opening I was so nervous I spent part of the time sitting on the bathroom floor. The show looked great, Stephanie sold all the work, and it was reviewed in *Artforum*. I am forever grateful to Stephanie and Carl. We bought one of Carl's paintings early on, paying him $100 a month, and it's always had a place of honor in our home.

Other shows and galleries followed. My work evolved and grew, and art was my life. I continued working temp jobs to support myself and I started doing a little adjunct teaching. And then, in 1999, we had our first child, followed by another two years later. When they were 9 months and 3 years old, we moved to St. Louis, where Paul had taken a job as director of a new museum, the Contemporary Art Museum St. Louis. I stopped working temp jobs since everything I earned would go directly to childcare. Paul was working all the time, traveling, spending time with supporters, and I was at home with two small children. I tried to paint after 9:00 p.m., once the kids were asleep, but after being up with them since 6:00 a.m., I just couldn't. I decided to stop beating myself up for not spending enough time painting and allow myself to relish these beautiful small people until they were old enough to be in preschool. That decision was one of the biggest gifts I ever gave myself, and I am so happy to have spent that time with them, without being too terribly conflicted. I still read a lot and looked at art a lot, did some small works, and took the kids to museums, galleries, and openings. St. Louis is a good art town, and the artists and art-supporters welcomed us. It was a good home.

By 2004 the kids were both in pre-school (for four hours a morning), and I found a nearby studio space. I would drop the kids off at school, do the five-minute drive to the studio, and leave the studio when it was time to pick the kids up. I rocked those four hours. It was pre-smart phone days. I didn't talk to anyone, I just worked. Fully focused work. From the first day back in the studio the work just flowed. I think I had been imagining working so much, visualizing the act of painting, and my body and mind just knew what to do. Yes, it was great to be back in the studio most days, and then it was also great to pick my kids up from school and be Mom.

After ten years in St. Louis, we moved to Boston in 2012 when another opportunity came along for Paul. The move was hard on the kids, as they didn't want to leave St. Louis, and if I had known how hard it would be on them I probably wouldn't have moved. But we wanted to be closer to our aging parents in Maryland, and it was also nice to be in a city with more museums, near the ocean, and in an environment where I could voice my political views a little more freely.

Always, when I'm not working, I'm thinking about when I can next be in the studio. When I'm not painting, I'm imagining painting. I think about what's in progress, and what the next steps are. Piled by my bed are art books and memoirs, another way of communing with artists here and gone. My mornings begin with me looking out the window as the sun rises and I say hello to the world, often followed by some solitary yoga or a walk, or just straight to the studio. Shows come and shows go, galleries come and galleries go. I don't feel the urgency to sell work like I did when I was younger and had to count my pennies in order to pay the rent. I make the work I want to make, following the twists and turns of "what if." A good thing about getting older is I don't care what other people think. My work has a right to exist, and yours does too.

I can remember sitting at my childhood desk, the one my father painted in bright colors for me, maybe I'm about 5, and I'm drawing, going round and round and round with a red crayon. I knew then that this was it, this was what I had to do. And it's the same feeling now, the feeling of oh my God this is what I want to do, I want to be an artist when I grow up. Having the place to make the work, with my tools nearby and the solitude I need, lets me pay full attention to the work at hand, so I can focus, be in the moment, and let the distractions and obligations fall away. It's the process of working more than the space itself that makes me feel all is right in my world, but the space allows the process to happen. This is what I'm supposed to do. I can just be. I am fortunate in that I am able to work in imperfect spaces. Spaces I have not looked forward to working in, spaces that depressed me when I anticipated walking into them, like the windowless basement in Soho where I painted right after our first child was born. But even when I've dreaded working somewhere, when the space has been kind of icky, dreary, or scary, I've found that as soon as I walk in knowing I will soon be working, knowing I'm in a space with time to work, the annoyances fall away, and I find myself in a world where my environment doesn't really matter. I start painting; I am happy to be there, it's where I want to be, in a room making thing.

There's still a lot of secrecy around money in the artworld, and plenty of artists who let us assume they're supported by their art when that's not really the case. I wish people would be more forthcoming. So here goes: Paul's career has provided financial stability, good health insurance, and retirement funding. But let's remember, it was my always being there for the kids that allowed him to work the long hours and travel, often with little notice. Paul could say, tomorrow I have to go to New York for three days, but I couldn't, as he was the breadwinner and if I left there would be no one to take care of the kids, because he still had to go to work.

It was hard for me, really hard, to have no family around when I was alone with the children, and I wished I had family nearby to invite me and the kids over for a casual dinner, or to take the kids for a night. Paul and I didn't plan for it to be that way, but that's what happened, and I guess you can call it teamwork of a sorts. Early on, Paul would take my slides for me, he made frames for me, helped me install shows, and would help pack and move my art. These days it's more an exchange of ideas, we're always texting each other articles, talking about what we think about shows, and the day-to-day nitty gritty of our work lives.

I don't doubt that Paul wished he had more time with the kids, and I know I wish I had more time in the studio these past twenty years. But I feel lucky that we are both in art, to share this beautifully consuming interest with my life partner. Our home is full of art made by friends, and art books are piled on the floor. Most of our friends are in art—artists, dealers, curators, and museum people—people who recognize art as essential, who build their lives around it, and who believe art talks about life with more accuracy and truth than anything else.

Now we're almost empty-nesters, and I am loving being able to stay in the studio longer, and not have to think about what will the kids eat for dinner, did I finish the paperwork for their school, blah blah blah. Money from art sales varies tremendously, and I teach part-time at the School of the Museum of Fine Arts at Tufts University so I can have some consistent income. Part-time teaching can easily start to feel full-time, and while I love working with young artists, I should be better about limiting the time I spend on my classes. And I learn from the students. Recently one of them said she has no interest in ever showing her work in a museum, and I was like, huh. Maybe her generation will come up with new ways of working and living as artists, and allow more good artists who don't have a support system or trust fund to thrive.

I get to live art, day in and day out. I read about art every day and look at friends' work on Instagram. I trade studio visits, and art too. The people I most want to hang out with are my family and art friends, so that's what I do. I think the pandemic taught us all to be a bit more choosey in who we spend our time with. Some of my best friends in Boston are artists whose parents are my age, and I'm so happy they welcome me into their lives.

Every time I walk into my studio I feel like I just won something. This is exactly where I want to be. •

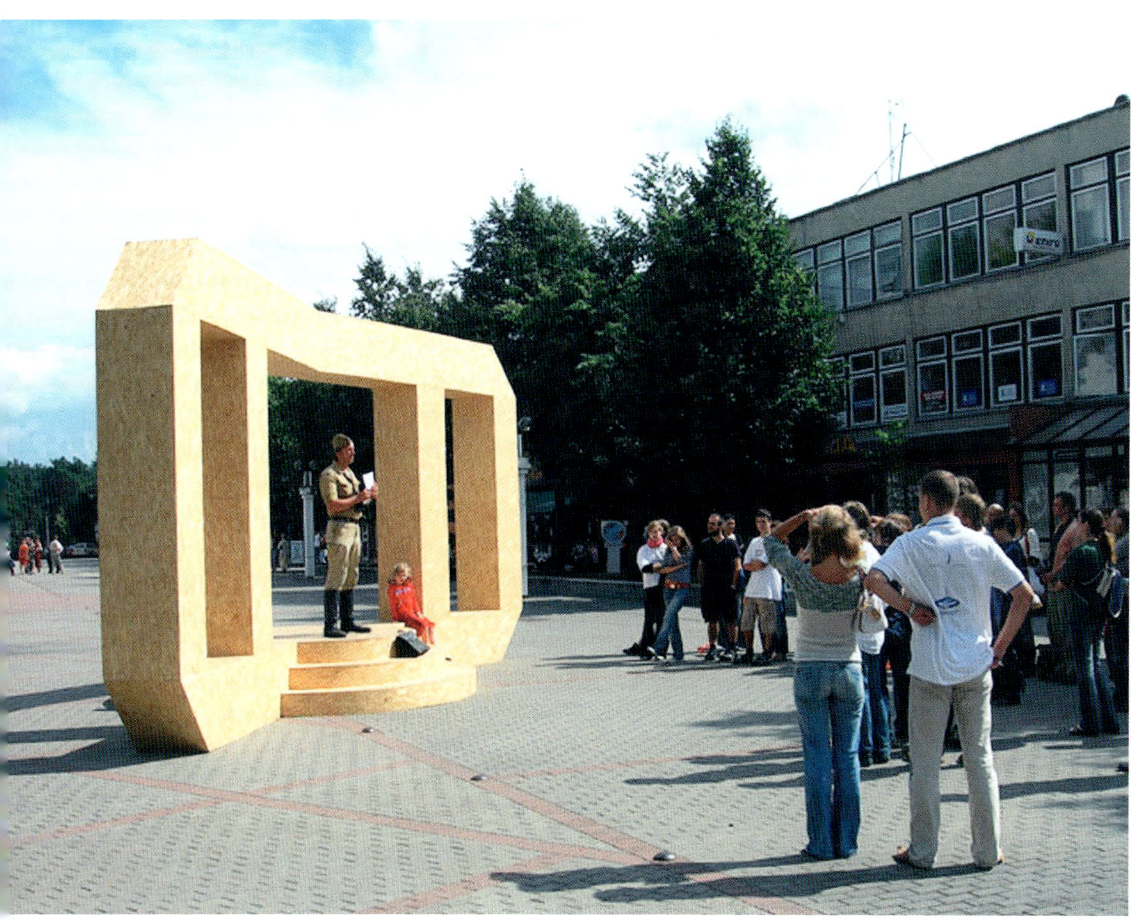

I AM AN African American artist. My culture is a byproduct of fate and geography. I grew up in the city of San Jose, in Northern California. During my upbringing, San Jose's Black population grew from around 1.0% of the city in 1960 to about 3.2% in 2010. There is no Black neighborhood in San Jose. There was no possibility for any African American to live a segregated life. My development as a person and as an artist evolved along two distinct paths.

One path chronicles my encounters within African American culture, and the other path critiques my journey through mainstream U.S. society. My local culture, the politics of my era, and my education, coalesce to shape the character of my person, and my art practice.

The Black people of San Jose did not exist in mass-media culture. Like other small and unique African-American communities, our modest humanity did not fit the "hip" archetype (stereotype) of the Black urban cauldron, like Harlem for example. The prevailing belief is authentic Black people hail primarily from the inner cities (the Ghetto). It is from within these communities that the globally dominant African American culture (music) emanates. Although we knew very well that our local mores failed to rise to the level of universal cultural distinction, we were clueless as to the determination that we may not be an "authentic" Black people.

Howard McCalebb
*Conjoined Icon / Edifice for Impromptu Theater (Alytus, Lithuania)*
2005
12'x 28'x 8'
Plywood
Courtesy of the artist

Our culture was a local phenomenon. We were the marginalized within the marginalized. When all the disparate African American communities merge (usually on college campuses), problems become exposed. There is a tendency for those from the most recognized group to speak and behave as if every Black person has the exact same culture—their culture. Within this heterogeneity, biracial Blacks may be insulted by undisciplined speech that disrespects their White, Mexican, Asian, or Jewish parents. There is variability within every population. No community is just one thing. The African American community is not one thing.

My family is atypical. I have a half-sister whose mother is Mexican. Five of my siblings married White people. Nearly twenty of my nieces, nephews, and cousins, are in interracial marriages of all kinds. One of my cousins has a White girl and boy as stepchildren, in addition to the two biracial boys he fathered with their mother. To paraphrase the Nigerian novelist Chimamanda Ngozi Adichie, who argued in a Ted Talk conference in July 2009: the significance of having a different story advocates for a greater respect for divergent experiences. By only understanding the single story (stereotype), one might misinterpret people, their background, their history, and their integrity.

San Jose is located about 45 miles south of San Francisco. In the 1960s, this region of California experienced dramatic developments in culture, politics, and technology, and an explosion of experimentation and innovation in fashion, music, and art. In 1967, activists, musicians, writers, and artists converged on the Haight-Ashbury neighborhood in San Francisco. Hordes of young people from all over the United States assembled there, including myself. I was encouraged by the atmospheric feeling that the world was changing for the better. I believed we were on the precipice of a truly just and equal society. That year marked the climax of the hippie movement. One of the momentous happenings was "The Summer of Love," a celebration of the counterculture that had blossomed there. The impetus to embrace women's liberation, ecological awareness, social justice, and a unified multiracial society was alive. Against the backdrop of the Vietnam War and the protests, activism became the ethos of our generation. This new attitude to life found its way into mainstream society. During the era of President Richard Nixon, Right-Wing Conservatives proclaimed loudly that the hippies would never contribute to society. Well ... look what happened. The hippies created the tech industry, which is the greatest economy in the history of mankind! This is a redeeming triumph of our generation. The tech industry (Silicon Valley) giants were some of the largest and most powerful companies in the world.

In 1966, I pursued my undergraduate education at California State University at Hayward (known today as Cal-State East Bay). I chose this school to bring myself closer to the San Francisco/Oakland Bay Area African American communities. An affirmative-action program was instituted in 1968; as a consequence, the Black student body at Cal-State Hayward increased, and became more militant. The priorities shifted; everything suddenly became about "the Ghetto, the Ghetto, the Ghetto." I began to feel that my racial bona fides were being interrogated—because I was from San Jose. I became defiant. Affirmative action also brought African American faculty to Cal-State Hayward for the first time. Previously there had been not one Black professor on the entire campus. Afterwards, the art department, and the African American professor Raymond Saunders, instituted a visiting artist program that brought artists from New York City to our school. Among them were some very important African American artists. These included Benny Andrews, Jacob Lawrence, William Majors, and Joe Overstreet. The influence of these artists inspired me to want to do graduate work on the East Coast, in or near New York City.

My art school education spans the ideological gamut between Northern California "Funk Art" and "The New York School." My serious foray into the art world began in earnest during my later years in undergraduate school. I started to frequent art galleries and museums regularly. A typical art school program is a situation where an older generation of artists foster their views and ideas upon a younger generation, where there might exist a chasm in ideology, a divergence of opinions, and a general evolution of social mores, etc. My generation eventually diverged onto our own path. We created and fortified our own language against outdated influences, to distinguish our ethos from that of the preceding tribe's (Hegel's Dialectical Negativity). We shifted out of the modes of late Modernist dogma, and solidified a Postmodernist critique. The most important gift of Postmodern art practice is that it eschews the constricting (Modernist) dogma of Reductionism. That alone was a great liberation!

I was accepted into the Cornell University College of Architecture, Art, and Planning Master of Fine Art (MFA) program. During my graduate studies at Cornell, from 1970 to 1972, I encountered writings by the artist Robert Motherwell, in the book *Robert Motherwell* by Frank O'Hara (1965). Le Corbusier's book *When the Cathedrals Were White* (1966) was another important read. To paraphrase Le Corbusier's philosophy, the solution to every problem begins with a proper statement of what the problem is. You cannot find a solution to a problem, if you do not state (understand) the problem correctly. For example: when a man said that he wanted to fly like a bird, every device and every attempt failed. The correct way to state the problem, to articulate the goal, was to say: I want to propel mass through air.

Airplanes do not fly like birds! Le Corbusier's insight can be instrumental, particularly when formulating strategies, for achieving the sociopolitical reforms Black activists have advocated for generations.

Immediately after graduate school, I taught art for five years at three different universities. Afterwards, I left teaching and moved to New York City to establish myself as a practicing artist. My art practice is conceived within the tumult of art world politics. I am resistant to what seems to be an identity politics mandate for African American artists. I challenge this dogmatic (lazy) imposition, by employing form and color as ideological devices. I configure my forms within a matrix created by the golden ratio, and I have reduced my general color palette to primary colors. Neither of these are the products of culture. Therefore, they hold no position within the dynamics of identity politics. I employ the golden ratio and the primary colors as "signifiers."

My generation came to ascendancy in the contemporary art world in the early 1980s. Sadly, the optimism engendered by the 1960s revolution was challenged by a counter force. Baby-Boomer utopia was counter attacked by a dystopian nightmare. My self-conceptualization was now being challenged on two fronts: The tyranny of Black identity politics and the neoconservative war on counterculture liberalism. African American activism during the 1960s, the advocacy for the Civil Rights Act, and the Black Power Movement, stimulated an anti-Black backlash in the form of the Neoconservative Political Movement. This group arose in the United States among people who shared a disdain for the counterculture. The "Neocons" as they are affectionately called, tend to pay an abnormal amount of attention to cultural matters, such as music, literature, theater, film, and the visual arts, because they believed that a society expresses its values through these agencies. Their position holds that multiculturalism will undermine Eurocentric culture in the United States. The Neocons exerted an influence in the mainstream art world to blunt the ascendancy of African American artists. Their aim was to stop social reform, or even to reverse social progress.

With regard to art world politics, I believe what is required of the individual artist is to measure one's commitment to progressive ideals. There are temptations to compromise one's integrity. Ambition, or even a survival tactic, may move some artists to become political sycophants. This penchant has given rise to the phenomenon of "Black Art for White People," which is a type of artwork steeped in racial stereotypes, that are employed for their powerful "sign" value. I refer to this type of artwork as (Ghetto) "Coon Art." With regard to my own art practice, I am cognizant of what I do, why I do it, and what are my inborn proclivities.

My life strategy going forward is to simply continue my art practice, and to persevere, over the course of my remaining years. I will manage to exist the best I can, especially within the continuing and difficult circumstances.

In 2022, I relocated to the United States after a long residence in Berlin, Germany. I have never married or had children.

I keep my life focused on my art practice, while also being flexible enough to improvise within life circumstances when necessary. One example would be my decision to move to Berlin, after being forced out of my TriBeCa loft by gentrification. Berlin was a cheap place to live and work at the time, so I simply moved there. It was just a move to survive. Nothing more, nothing less. ●

# JAMES CLARK

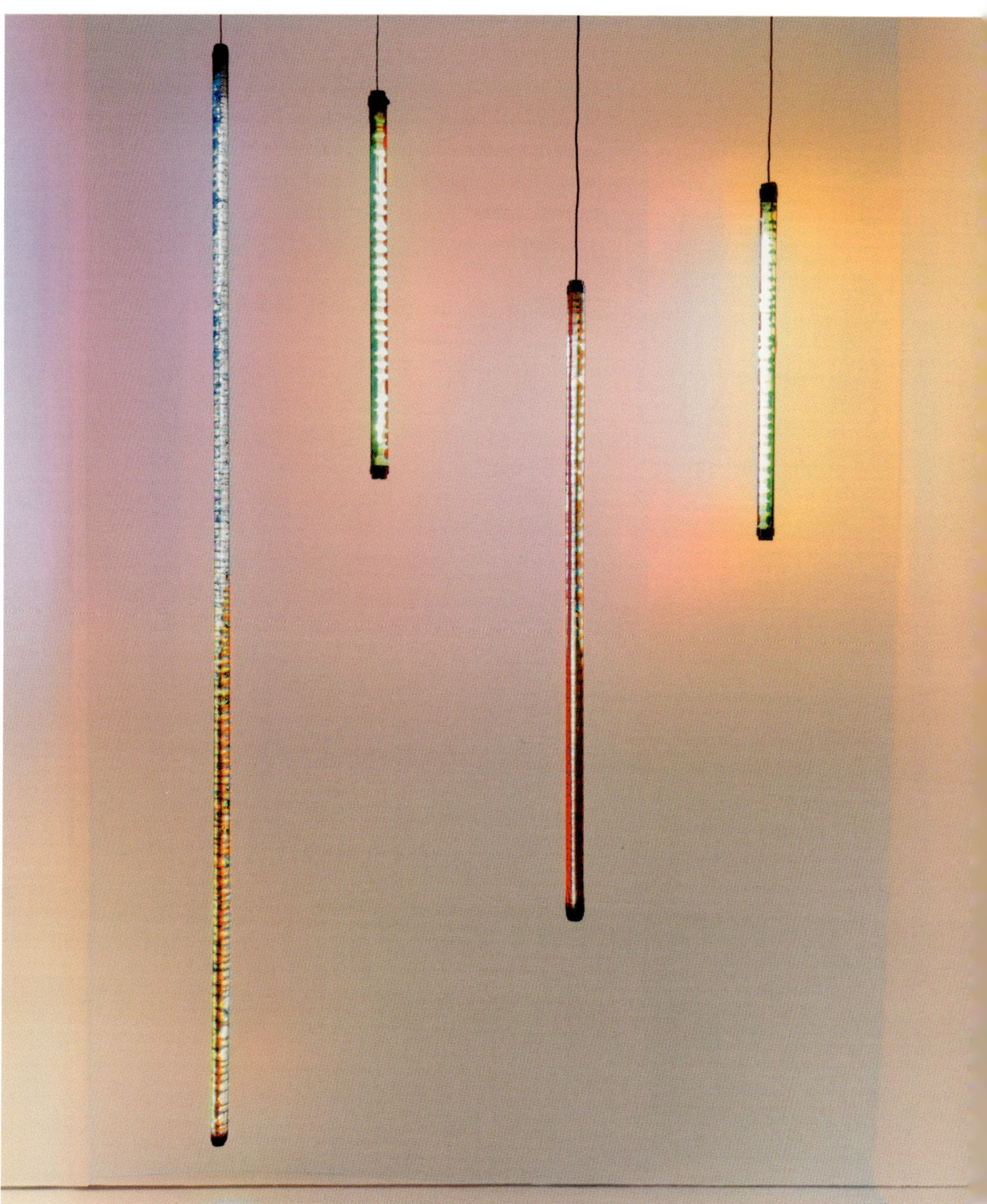

James Clark
*Augenwiede*
2022
92″(h)x68″(w)x19″(d)
Epoxy pigment, polycarbonate tubes, LED cob lights
Courtesy of the artist and Studio Rondinone
Photography by Francisco Ramirez Barrera

IN 1954, at the age of 6, I got bitten by a bug: The Art-Bug. I found that art got into my being; why it was there I can never understand nor what path in life I would travel. I lived with my mother and father, who worked in the steel mill, near the small steel town of Coatesville, Pennsylvania. After my mother died in 1954, my father and I moved to Cochranville, Pennsylvania. My memories of where I lived were romantic, filled with freedom, beautiful rolling hills, lavish green landscapes—a visual playground filled with light, space, and the best was the evening with lightning bugs. I navigated the landscape on foot, bicycle, or traveled by vehicle; the rural way of life.

I reminisced, looking out the window while riding inside the car with the light illuminating interior and exterior space, giving my eyes the invitation to explore the content and the context of the passing forms. Light felt like magic, and it was the center of my universe, my life's energy. It seemed to have a language of its own, speaking in many tones and volumes with endless musical abstractions that I could see and hear growing up, and still do today.

A nighttime imprint for me is remembering light crystals on fallen snow and the Northern Lights (Aurora Borealis). These are but a few of nature's many environmental light shows which created visual wonderments. Light as a material has illuminated my creative search from early on.

My first theatrical experience with light was observing the light that hung over the billiards table in a recreation room at the Cochranville Fire House in 1960. Over the years, in my creative search, light has been my driving force.

Being in this locale, cars were a status symbol. I remember lights under the wheel wells reflecting off the hubcaps. I remember that like it was yesterday and try to catch that moment in my work.

In 1964, my father died. I was shuffled around to different schools and living situations. I was trying to fit in with different groups and doing odd jobs.

In 1966, I graduated from Coatesville High School. After graduating, I worked on computers at Borroughs Corporation until I was drafted into the Army. The computers were so large, I would walk inside of them to do the wiring.

In 1968, I was drafted into the Army. My basic training was at Fort Bragg in Fayetteville, North Carolina. I was transferred to Fort Hood in Killeen, Texas. While I was in Killeen, I often went to Austin, Texas, to the Vulcan Gas Company where they played music and had light shows. I remember the multi-colored posters for the concerts. After less than two years in the army, I got an early out to go to Pierce Junior College, majoring in business management, in Philadelphia, Pennsylvania. During the summer of 1970, I got a full-time job working as a brakeman on the Reading Railroad in Coatesville, Pennsylvania. My responsibilities were to classify and shift heavy steel plates at Lukens Steel Mill. I was able to transfer my position on the Reading Railroad to Philadelphia in order to pay my tuition.

I was getting pressured by my family to go into medicine. So in the fall of 1971, I transferred my Reading Railroad job back to Coatesville and enrolled at West Chester State College to major in biology. While in the lab viewing a slide through the microscope, I had an aesthetic epiphany. I interrupted the class to share my visual excitement about the forms and colors on the slide. The teacher said, "You know Jim, everyone has the same forms and colors on their slide." She said, "You don't belong in the biology department. You belong in the art department." I responded, "You're right." I immediately went to the art department and said, "I want to transfer." All through this period, I continued to work full time on the Reading Railroad. While shifting heavy freight loads of scrap and finished plate steel. I gathered various pieces of metal in different forms from machine stampings. My earliest sculptures were made from these findings.

In winter 1971, massive ingots were brought out from the steel mill furnace. Glowing neon red/orange, they were so hot that snow was melting in their proximity. I can still flash back to many amazing moments of color, light, mass, and movement. That environment deeply affected my creativity in the studio.

As an art student at West Chester State College, I met the sculptor/professor Billy Neumann. Billy was my first art mentor who had a large footprint in my early development as an artist. He shared his artwork with me, introduced me to the artist Harry Bertoia and his sculptures, and urged me to transfer to Kutztown State College to work with the sculptor/professor/author James J. Kelly.

In fall 1972, I transferred to Kutztown State College. I was still working on the Reading Railroad. While I was a student at Kutztown, I was fortunate to work with James J. Kelly, a hands-on sculptor who had an encyclopedic knowledge about materials. I experienced pouring aluminum bronze sculptures while working with him. James Carroll was another professor at Kutztown who is a force to be reckoned with, is James Carroll. James created the Visiting Artist Program which was the creme-de-la-creme, challenging young creative minds. I was exposed to a variety of artworks and mediums as well as artists with different visions. It was my first introduction to artists that were living and working in the New York area.

Over that period, I made lifelong friendships that pulled me into creating art within an art community. Gary Stephan, Kent Floeter, Richard Serra, Paula Cooper, Phil Glass, and Dorothea Rockburne were among the many artists that James Carroll invited to participate in the Visiting Artists Program that created an impact on my life, supportive to my work and education. It was a great time to expand my views of the integration and assimilation of different technologies into my art and confirmed my decision to move to New York City.

In 1973, while still a student at Kutztown, I met my future wife Linda outside the sculpture studio. I was immersed in my art but I remember her blue eyes and positive energy like it was yesterday. I was also working part time with the Gretz sign company, installing neon and fluorescent light advertising. In 1974, after graduating from Kutztown with a Bachelor of Science (BS) in art education, I worked for Earl Smith roofing company for six months repairing and replacing metal and shingle roof surfaces.

By the mid-1970s, my experiences from work were being incorporated into my creativity. In 1976, I worked again on the railroad as a track man, laying steel rails and ties, hammering spikes, and working with large heavy equipment. It was a completely different experience to work outside in the landscape and within nature. This was a very important period, seeing a quarter mile of ribbon steel rail cushioned by stone as a ballast, mass holding mass together. At this point, I was a human sponge trying to grow and abstractly express my creative search.

In 1977, I made the most important decision of my life: I moved to New York City to pursue a career as an artist and to join a community of like-minded creative individuals. It was difficult to find an affordable space to live and work. In order to survive, I worked construction jobs and as an assistant to the artist Lucio Pozzi. Within six months, I converted and was evicted from three studios. After walking from SoHo to TriBeCa to the Lower East Side, one day I stopped in a used appliance store on Delancey Street. The guy suggested I talk to Frankie on 250 South Street. He said he may have space available. Frankie was a trucker who had a trucking business, and 250 South Street was an empty building that he wanted to rent out. The building had no windows, holes through the roof, no plumbing, and no electricity. Basically it was a wide-open shell. I rented 2,000 square feet for $100 a month. Other artists soon moved into the building, including Bill Jensen, Margrit Lewczuk, and Kiki Smith.

In summer 1977, while doing construction work, I fell off a ladder and shattered my elbow. Linda, my friend and future wife, visited me in the hospital. After seeing my physical condition she said she would move to New York to help me. After I was discharged from the hospital in late summer '77, Linda moved to New York City. Soon after her arrival, we were robbed, by gunpoint, in front of our live-work studio. Our families wanted us to leave the city, but I wanted to be true to my art and stay in New York City.

In 1978, Jensen encouraged me to share a studio building in Williamsburg, Brooklyn, with him and the sculptor Robert Grosvenor. I rented 3,500 square feet for $80 a month. During this period, I met the sculptors Ronald Bladen, Forrest Myers, and Mark di Suvero. These creators, with their deeply dedicated approach to art-making, left a large footprint in my life. These relationships were unique because these artists were role models, offered guidance, inspiration, were very generous, supportive of my artistic journey, and they were an important factor in the development of my career. I learned from these masters that these values should be shared.

In 1983, my wife and I found ourselves without a home and I without a studio. I diligently searched for hours, day in and day out. I finally found a neglected and vulnerable structure, which at the time was in a risqué neighborhood with drugs, gangs, sex workers, etc., also in Williamsburg.

I looked at this diamond in the rough and had the most incredible vision: the spirit emanating from this building called to me. The way it perched on the cityscape with its own timeless integrity. As the morning sun greets the rear of the building and the sunset warms the front entrance, highlighting all the architectural details, one can only imagine the moments of time when children played in the courtyard bathed in nature's sunlight. I knew deep in my heart that this was meant to be our home and my studio. When I brought Linda to look at the building she asked, "Can you make art here? Because, I can't live with you if you can't make art." Even though this hundred-plus year-old structure was tattered and torn, it was like a newborn baby to us, needing all our tender loving care. We were young and lovingly blind to the enormous project we would encounter. Physically, emotionally, and spiritually this building became our light. We felt and still feel blessed with the ownership of this property, even today. But we are in fact, just temporary caretakers. While this property has its roots in the past, it reflects an optimistic and visual future for generations.

In renovating and restoring 270 Union Avenue, Linda and I had to live apart for a year because there was no plumbing, no heat, no windows, no security, etc. The building had good bones but no systems. After a year, we were able to live in the basement as we worked on the rest of the building.

In 1986, I was invited to mentor work term students at Bennington College. Each year a student would live with us for two months and do interior renovation. One student, James Sadek, returned several times to share the vision. By the mid-1980s, Williamsburg was changing. Two very important sculptors, Judy Pfaff and Ursula Von Rydingsvard, became my neighbors and friends.

The year 1989 was a milestone year for me. Artist David Reed introduced me to his dealer Max Protetch and I had a one-person show at the Protetch Gallery in May. I also received a Guggenheim Fellowship. In the summer of 1989, I was asked to teach at the Skowhegan School of Painting and Sculpture, where I met the painter John Walker.

In September 1989, our daughter, Tessa was born. Tessa opened up a whole new dimension in my existence. Watching her development in all its stages opened up new visual intelligence for my work. Her birth was the beginning of the magical journey of life. Her innocence and freshness challenged my artistic sensibilities in dimensions I never could have imagined. I made a series of work that included soft materials against more industrial hard materials, which was a big shift in my work. When Tessa was about 5, she asked me to make a pink and purple sculpture. This was a challenge to my sensibility and Tessa was a tough critic.

In 1990, I had a one-person exhibition at Seibu in Tokyo, Japan followed by a second one-person show at Max Protetch in 1991. My exhibition had the most reviews the gallery had ever received in 25 years. Although it was well received critically, there were no financial rewards. I continued working in the studio and doing construction with the sculptor Tom Bills, to survive. We also had some income from Linda's teaching.

In 1993, I was highlighted in an article in the Sunday *New York Times Magazine* titled "The Art World Bust." At the time, I was doing construction for the artist Yoko Ono. When I was interviewed, the author wanted me to be photographed in Yoko Ono's studio holding a wrench in my hand. I had previously been photographed in my studio standing with my daughter and my sculptures. I said, "I am a sculptor. There's a big difference in what one does and what one is." I stated, "If the photograph of my daughter and I in my studio is not good enough; I want no parts of your article."

From 1994–99, I was a visiting artist at many colleges, including Vermont Studio Center, Brown University, Boston University, and Bennington College.

In 1999, I was nominated by Marthe Keller as a member of American Abstract Artists. I also had a one-person installation exhibition at Nicholas Davies titled *Tulips Hysteria Coordinating*. This title was from a painting that Marcel Duchamp was supposed to place in the *First Annual Exhibition* in 1917. My installation was well received.

In 2000, I was approached to teach a sculpture class at Princeton University. I had the good fortune to meet the artists James Seawright (who was a pioneer in Electronic Art and head of the university's art department) and Creighton Michael. Creighton is a dedicated creator who is still very generous in his support for other artists and a wealth of historical information.

From 2000–11, I continued to be a visiting artist at different universities, do construction work, and also taught at Brandeis, Bard, and University of Connecticut.

During these years, my work was in multiple shows and was included in some important exhibitions. At this point in time, I had been in NYC for over 25 years and I had a well-developed support base of artists, writers, and critics that promoted my work. This happens naturally by being present in a community of like-minded creators who share the same values, fostering reciprocation, which brings people more together.

In 2006, my work was shown with Tara Donovan at Maier Museum of Art. In 2011, I showed in an exhibition titled *Luminous Flux* with Forrest Myers ("Frosty") at Regina Rex Gallery curated by Heather Hubbs, the director of The New Art Dealers Alliance (NADA). Frosty is an innovative creator. I had been aware of his work since the 1970s and was honored my work was included in a two-person exhibition with him.

In 2009, I did an installation at the Lesley Heller Gallery titled *Poultry in Motion*. This was an outdoor installation, and I was given total freedom to display live tie-dyed chickens. One bird had a camera affixed to its back to livestream the opening on a wall. I created an interactive environment with a fur-coated singing fish, bubbles, mist, fiber optics, and manufactured odor that engaged the viewer. This installation made me stretch outside my comfort zone using all of my sensory perceptions. This exhibition somehow has legs going beyond the presentation, standing the test of time.

In 2012, the painter Jake Berthot recommended me to take his MFA graduate class at the School of Visual Arts. I was given freedom to put my ideas into action. In teaching my classes, I think about what I would have wanted as a student; having students hold a mirror up for self-examination, and following the wisdom of the sculptor and Head of the Sculpture Department at Yale, David von Schlegell, "Listen, talk about materials, talk about historical roots and let them find themselves."

In 2015, I was invited to build an installation for an exhibition at the ltd Gallery in Los Angeles. Instead of bringing my work with me, I repurposed the existing fluorescent lights in the ltd Gallery itself to create the work. As viewers entered the gallery space, the motion sensors would be triggered by their presence; turning the pieces off and on.

My most recent exhibition of my work was a show that traveled from 1993–2020. It was curated by T. Michael Martin, who was introduced to my work by Creighton Michael. Jonathan Lippincott, a respected critic and author, wrote the essay. This show has traveled to three different venues and is scheduled to be presented in the New York City area in 2025. Through my lifelong relationships with artists, writers, poets, collectors, dealers, students, critics, and just people I meet in my life exchanges and the global community; we organically connect, support, and recommend one another and that still occurs today.

I believe that my relationships that start with mentoring students continue as they become artists and therefore a part of my world.

As an artist I am very fortunate to be able to share my work, have a studio/home, have a family including my daughter Tessa, great friends, and a wife that believes in me. Linda is a guiding light being finely tuned to my creative search and artistic adventure for the past 50 years. I am thankful to have such a partner. ●

# JAQ CHARTIER

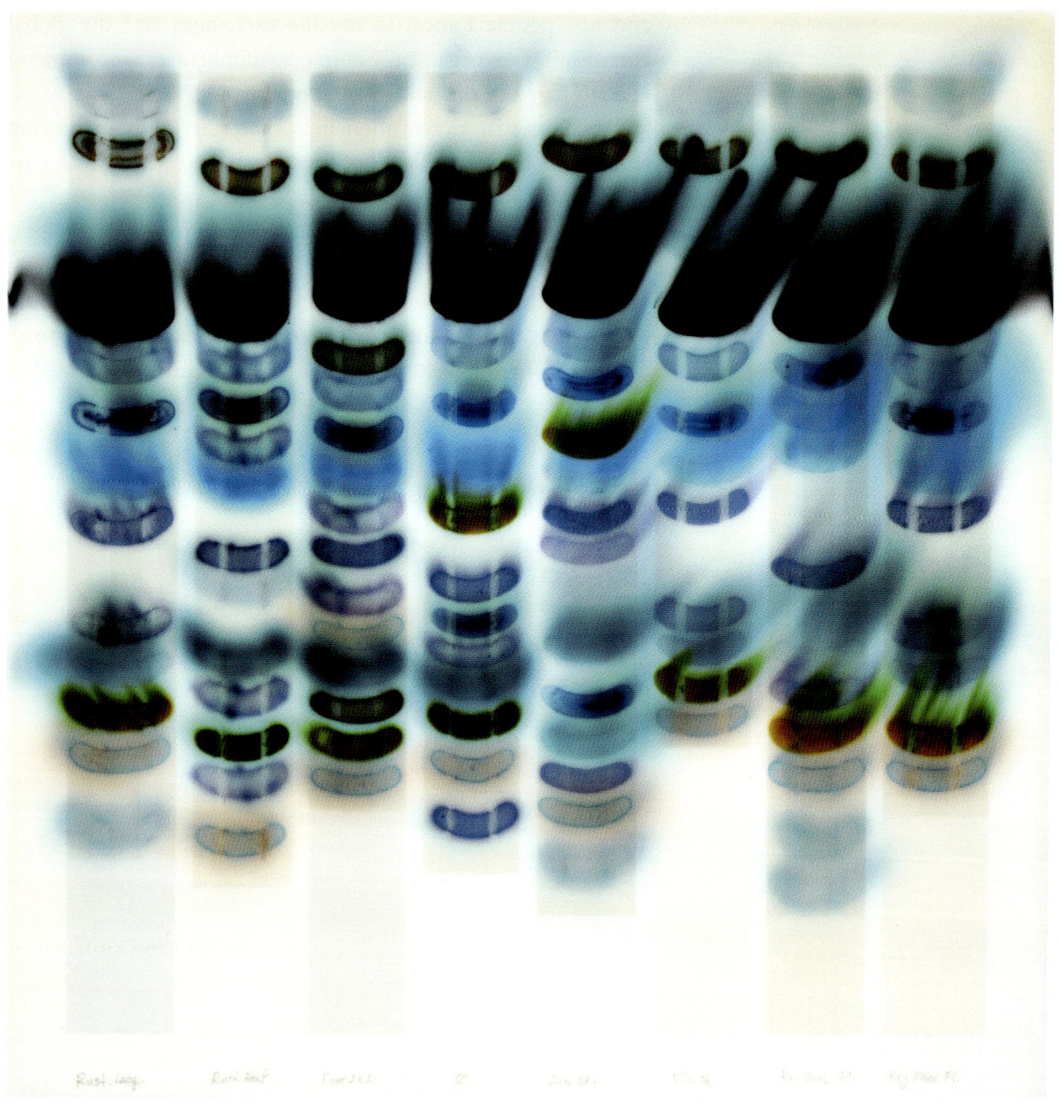

I STARTED painting when I was around 12 years old, inspired by my mom who also liked to paint. Three years later, I was fortunate to go to Palmer High School in Palmer, Massachusetts, which had an unusually substantial art program for such a small town. After graduation I went to Syracuse University in New York to study filmmaking. It took me a few semesters to realize I wanted to be a painter for real—and for that kind of career, I thought it would be best not to have a lot of student-loan debt. My mom was working at the University of Massachusetts, Amherst, where tuition would be free for me, so I transferred into their painting program.

After getting my BFA from UMass in 1984, I spent the bulk of my twenties in the nearby Northampton area, a hub for music, art, and progressive culture. I worked in an art store and continued to paint, and just lived my life for a while.

Eventually I was ready for the focused rigor of grad school and moved to Seattle to study painting at the University of Washington. It was the summer of 1992 and the city's music scene was on fire. I was a huge Nirvana fan and it was the music that drew me across the country. My then-husband Tim Gabor was an illustrator and willing to move anywhere that had access to FedEx. My first glimpse of the city from I-90 was thrilling and anything seemed possible. It would have stunned me to know that just a few years later, Kurt Cobain (of Nirvana) would be dead, his bandmate Dave Grohl would come to my MFA

Jaq Chartier
*Blues w/8 Whites*
2020
16″x16″
Acrylic, inks, dyes, stains & spray paint on wood panel
Courtesy of the artist

thesis show, and my paintings would end up on the first album for Dave's new band the Foo Fighters, which would become superstars.

Meeting Dave Grohl was pure luck. While I was studying at the University of Washington, one of my close grad school buddies, Martha Parrish Bush, had a side job cleaning houses—which ended up including Dave's house and Krist Novoselic's (Nirvana's bass player) house. She wasn't really a Nirvana fan, so she was unfazed by their fame and became friends with their wives. She invited them all to our MFA thesis exhibition opening a month after Kurt Cobain died, thinking they probably wouldn't come. But Dave and his wife, Jennifer, actually showed up to support Martha.

My minimal paintings had a UFO vibe that caught Dave's eye and we became friends. I didn't get the full significance of his response to my work until a few months later at dinner when Dave handed Tim and me a cassette tape and said he was starting a band called the Foo Fighters (a type of UFO). Dave asked if he could include my work on his album and if Tim would design the whole package. Later in the car on the way home we popped in the demo tape and realized this new band was going to be a huge success.

Meanwhile, it was 1994, I was out of grad school and needed a studio. I had taken a chunk of time between undergrad and grad school, and knew things could get bleak back out in the real world. Friends would soon scatter if we all didn't do something about it, so we banded together and started hunting for a space to share in Seattle.

Martha and I finally found a 4,200 square-foot basement space for $1,200 per month in a light industrial building that was under renovation. I put together a floor plan, the landlord's crew built the stud walls, and the group of us figured out the rest together.

Although it started as a co-op and ran that way for a while, eventually one and then another of the founding group moved away. I had been the one who signed the lease (because I co-owned a gargoyle statuary store, another story!)—so I ended up managing the space. When the ground floor became available I grabbed it for more studios, and then another floor. Each time it felt risky and was a big stretch out of my comfort zone. But it also made practical sense that I turn this into a job, getting a free studio and some income out of the deal. I signed long leases and kept renewing. Over the years more than 200 artists passed through that building, many of whom are still friends. Twenty-five years later when the building was sold, they bought me out of my lease and I got a chunk of money to invest in another way.

Collaborations have been the heart and soul of so many interesting projects in my life, and have set new chains of events in motion. Managing the studios led to organizing open-studio events with the artists in my building. At some point I thought, why not a city-wide open studios event? In 1999, I teamed up with artists in other studio buildings around the city and we created Art Detour Seattle, a city-wide open studios weekend event. It was a ton of work and we could only sustain it for a few years before hitting burnout, but I learned so much.

While we were building out our post-grad studios, my cohorts Martha, Carol Bolt, and Katy Stone were also co-founding a gallery with some other friends called SOIL, which is still one of the best artist-run galleries anywhere. I met my now-husband Dirk Park through his membership in SOIL. Later on, Dirk and Carol teamed up with some other artists to create a commercial gallery called Platform. And when they wanted to bring Platform to Miami Beach during the week of Art Basel Miami Beach art fair, we thought starting our own satellite art fair seemed reasonable.

I like to say I accidentally founded an art fair, like accidentally having a baby. It started with a little flirty idea while talking with my art dealer, Elizabeth (Liz) Leach. It was in the fall of 2004 and we were at a small art fair in Portland, Oregon, called Affair at the Jupiter Hotel. The Jupiter was a chic, U-shaped space with 2 floors of rooms opening out to a central courtyard filled with plants and party lights. I had been to Art Basel week in Miami Beach, because another of my galleries had brought my work to the fledgling New Art Dealers Alliance (NADA) art fair. The two events merged in my mind and I said to Liz, "wouldn't it be cool if we could find a hotel like this in Miami Beach and bring a bunch of west coast galleries?" Her eyes got big and she got it right away. "HELL YES!!"

A few months later, Dirk and I were back in Miami Beach again for Art Basel week and on the hunt. I distinctly remember at one point saying, "If it had a courtyard we'd see palm trees poking up over the roofline, kind of like that—" as I pointed at the Aqua Hotel. The woman at the front desk was our first supporter and let me take a ton of photos inside many rooms. Cement floors, minimal furniture, a breezy courtyard with lush plants and a hot tub. We could totally see it. I gave her my credit card to hold it for us for next year.

Once we returned home, we started asking Seattle art dealers if they were interested and everyone we spoke with said yes immediately. The moment was just right. Our heads were swirling with all the details of putting an art fair together from scratch—and, yes, we were scared shitless! But we were all in. We knew the mothership Art Basel Miami Beach art fair that attracted top collectors and curators from around the world. Aqua was just a short walk away, so the odds were good that West Coast artists and galleries would be on the world stage. And suddenly we all were!

Dirk and I co-directed Aqua for eight years, ultimately selling it to a bigger fair. At times it was a trial by fire, but it was also a lot of fun, and now I feel like I can handle just about anything.

I think I got my entrepreneurial backbone from my mom. She was an unconventional feminist and single parent with a hardcore do-it-yourself spirit. Although money was tight, she taught me that you can always make things a little better by noticing what you have access to and putting in some effort.

In 1971, when I was 10 years old, we moved into a run-down tenement building in Three Rivers, a tiny village that's part of Palmer, Massachusetts, where my mom's family lived. The landlord owned a hardware store, so my mom arranged for free supplies and organized the neighbors to help us paint all the porches and trim and plant flowers. It lifted everyone's spirits while building a sense of community in what would have been a dreary place otherwise. She decorated our rooms with thrift-store furniture painted all the same color so it felt new. My sister's room was all shiny lavender enamel, a lime green shag rug, and purple wallpaper with gold flecks.

My brother, sister, and I were her little helpers in these and other creative projects to bring in extra cash. My mom was transparent about money and all the business ups and downs, so we could learn what worked and what didn't. She was also my earliest supporter as a budding artist, and I could write pages about those crucial years early on. Because of her, I've lived a happy life gathering what's at hand and shaping something new from it, both in the studio and in my life. I miss her dearly.

In another lucky chain of events, my work ended up on the Showtime television show *Billions*, and on the wall of the Microsoft headquarters in Seattle.

Erica Behrens, the New York director of Mayer of Munich glass fabricator, visited my studio and suggested I try working in glass, which I hadn't been thinking about at all. We became fast friends and her enthusiasm for glass took root in my mind. Meanwhile, I noticed a social media post by Lele Barnett, then-curator for Microsoft's art collection, and invited her for a studio visit. That led to a big glass commission for Microsoft, fabricated by Mayer of Munich, which launched the public art wing of my career. A few years later, Erica was invited to curate a list of artists for consideration for season four of "Billions", and I ended up being one of the artists chosen. People have asked how I got that gig—because we're all trying to figure out the secret sauce. But what are the odds? I say my mom was pulling strings from the great beyond!

Over the years I've nearly always had more than one gallery representing my work. Most have been outside of the major art scenes of New York, Los Angeles, etc., but it's worked out pretty well, and I've made a decent living from my studio for a long time. I've also lost some galleries along the way, and those moments could have been soul crushing. A few cases were pretty bad—not being paid for sold work, passive-aggressive behavior and other shell games. But one benefit of having more than one gallery was that I could compare behavior and get some perspective on what was happening. Each of my current dealers has become a trusted friend and I'm so grateful for them. They are hardworking and brave entrepreneurs, true champions of their artists in a tough business. They give me room to work at my slow-burn pace, which I'm sure is maddening for them at times, and they remain supportive no matter what.

I'm also grateful for my friends, who bring their talent, humor, and wisdom to every conversation. About seven years ago, I formed a group called "Asskickers." Getting together over cocktails, we talk about what's happening in our careers, the good and the bad. Sometimes it's about setting goals for things that would help our careers if we just took the steps. Other times it's about celebrating each other's accomplishments.

My luckiest break was meeting my husband Dirk Park. He has a keen eye and lots of good ideas, which gets me out of my studio bubble and into the world (sometimes). Together we've built various creative businesses and have been completely self-employed for a number of years.

I recently renewed a second 10-year lease on my current studio in downtown Seattle, where we also built out additional art studio sublets and added an Airbnb unit. We also own a small apartment that we bought when we sold the Aqua fair, which is also a lucrative Airbnb. I manage the studios, which affords me a great deal on my own space, and I'm in my studio nearly every day, while Dirk does most of the Airbnb work. This combo works for us financially, and gives us flexibility to take time off as needed.

A lot of this wouldn't have been possible if not for the affordable rent at the Tashiro Kaplan Artist Lofts in Seattle's downtown Pioneer Square neighborhood, where we've lived for nearly twenty years. The building was restored by Artspace, a nonprofit arts organization specializing in developing affordable spaces for artists in cities around the country. Though the neighborhood is transitional and a bit rough at times, it includes a lot of art galleries and other creative venues, it's very diverse, and provides a dynamic urban experience. I love living right in the city, but for a lot of other artists it's becoming nearly impossible to afford.

Seattle's art scene is gradually recovering after nearly three years of the COVID-19 pandemic, but things still feel muted and fragile. Like many artists around the globe, most of my recent shows and other achievements have happened in a kind of void due to social distancing, some without opening receptions, or taking place out of town without the ability to travel there. It's been a strange time. I've stayed connected with galleries, collectors, artists and other associates through social media, and we've supported each other in other ways when we couldn't be there in the flesh. Those personal connections are the bedrock of my art community. It all builds from there.

# JENNIFER WEN MA

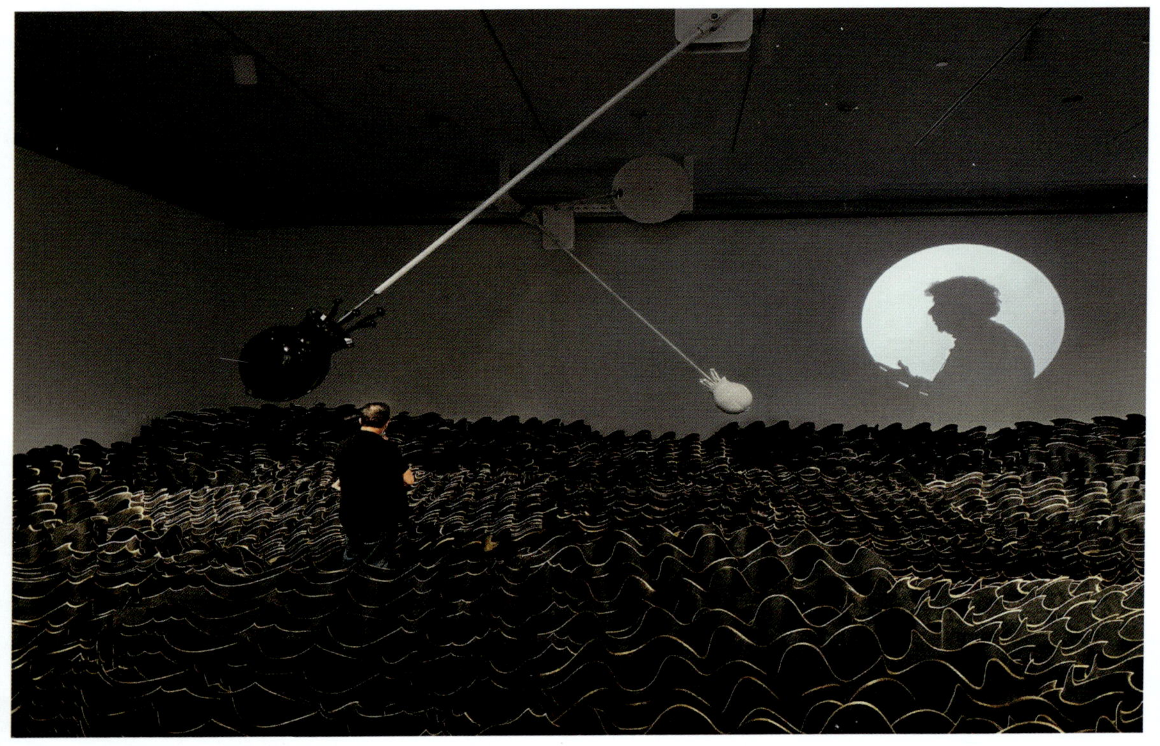

GROWING UP I wanted to be a writer. When I was 12, I moved from Beijing, China, to Edmond, Oklahoma, in the summer of 1986. Verbal and written communication became the biggest source of frustration in my daily life. I took an art class to have an easy period in school and fell into drawing and painting, finding a world without a language barrier and a new mode of expression. I wonder what creative path I might have taken had I stayed in China. I no longer identify with writing; the process of contributing to this book has shown me that I am still not a comfortable writer. It seems creativity, resilience, and adaptation found an alternative route to channel through me.

## WENDY'S RESERVOIR

In 2000, I went to my local bank to do a simple transaction. I sat down in front of a financial advisor, Wendy, who told me that I needed to open a savings account. I was not convinced, fresh out of graduate school with tens of thousands of dollars in student-loan debt and working at a low-wage art job, I had zero money to spare. But Wendy assured me that I would not miss the money, which would be automatically transferred to the new savings account at the first of each month, and I could use the funds for something that was truly important in the future. I started with $50, and six months later came back to increase it to $200. She was right, I didn't miss it. In the subsequent

Jennifer Wen Ma
*An Inward Sea*
2021
Dimensions variable
Laser-cut flashspun non-woven HDPE, pigments, glass sculptures, metal mechanisms, video, and audio tracks
Courtesy of the artist

years, every time I got a raise or promotion, that savings account did too.

In 2007, I made the decision to devote the best hours of each day to making my art, instead of assisting another artist's career. It meant leaving the stability of a regular paycheck. But I had Wendy's reservoir to draw from. I paid off my student debt and had enough savings to live frugally in NYC for two years without additional income. I was committed to giving myself the time to develop work without financial pressure.

Over the years, I have continued to draw from that reservoir for the most important projects. I have also made efforts to re-invest into it for future dreams. An artist's life means being in a constant state of feast or famine. Living, budgeting, saving, and investing smartly has been foundational to my financial sustainability. I learned through Wendy that no amount is too small to begin that practice.

## TO THE RAVINE

Twenty-five years ago when I was a young artist, I met France Morin, a renowned curator. I admired her work and sought her out as a friend and mentor, wanting an ally who was senior and could shed light on my artistic path as I developed—a perspective that my peers wouldn't be able to provide. I offered my energy and youth in a friendship that took years to build; slowly, we became important people in each other's lives.

In 2009, I started a new series of work, applying Chinese to live plants to create all-black tableaux that would grow and change with time. About a year into it, while discussing the work with France, she sensed my reservation and said, "Jennifer, you must go all in. Art will take you to the edge of the cliff, and you look into the depth of the fall and jump—there is no holding back! To the ravine!"

I went on to make a six-ton garden suspended in midair, an island in the center of a lake, and a rotating asteroid, among other projects. Now this is my rallying cry whenever I feel scared and unsure about a new work. I say to myself, "Courage! To the ravine! To the ravine!" I am all in, ready to leap and fly.

## MY FATHER'S DOUBTS

My parents belonged to the first generation of computer hardware engineers in China, contributing to prestigious national projects. When they first moved to the United States in the 1980s, they took many jobs—nanny, housekeeper, dishwasher—before finding their professional footing. They made these sacrifices to forge new paths for themselves and provide better opportunities for my brother and me.

Art was not their envisioned trajectory for a better future. In 1989, when I enrolled in the art and design program at Oklahoma Christian University, they were skeptical: "we sacrificed everything so you could draw all day?!" They worried about the uncertainty of this career path. Additionally, my father, who has a deep sense of social responsibility, couldn't see how such a seemingly self-centered practice could contribute to the betterment of mankind.

Upon my graduation in 1993, I had decided not to pursue design as a profession, but to become an artist. My parents disapproved and began a grueling pressure campaign to redirect me toward a more practical profession. But I was as bullheaded as they were and persisted on my meandering path toward art making.

In 2005, I produced the inaugural China Pavilion at Venice Biennale, and invited my parents to the opening festivities. Everything went exceptionally well, from the artworks to the press conference and opening parties. Each event we hosted drew a full audience, from diplomats, to artworld luminaries and the press.

The impact of an art event's ability to attract people worldwide and influence a city and region left a profound impression on my father. Beyond the glamour and glitz, he was moved by the passion and meaning that artists infused into their work. My parents became vested in the China Pavilion project that centered on a self-made flying object by a Chinese farmer brought to Venice by the artists' team for the opening performance.

As lifelong engineers, my parents' eagle eyes saw that the design was flawed from the start, that the engine would never enable the structure to fly. But they said nothing and were even nervous for the artists. They understood the significance of this attempt—a farmer, who never had formal training in engineering or aerodynamics, attempting to fly an object of his own design and construction, and the foolhardy artists who poured all their resources to enable this act, for the first official participation of China in the preeminent contemporary art event of the world.

The Venice Biennale experience changed my parents' perspective of the value of an art worker's vocation. They were persuaded by the seriousness of this work and its potential impact. To this day my dad thoughtfully reads curatorial and artistic statements from each of my projects and would ask to meet for a discussion. He brings questions and comments, sometimes puzzlement, sometimes pride, sometimes with tears in his eyes.

The path to being an artist is hard, there are some who don't wish us well, and many more who don't care. Having lived through sixteen years of opposition that was rooted in love made me stronger. I had the deep conviction that I was on the art path for the long haul, and eventually I would win over my family and the world.

## BE A FRIEND MAKE A FRIEND

When I meet an artist whose work I like, I make an effort to tell them what I like about it and why. I ask them to lunch or tea. I offer to visit their studio and welcome them to mine. If we are like minded, I share information and resources, invite them to collaborate on a project or opportunity, and check in regularly. I have cultivated a wonderful and supportive network of friends in the arts that help me thrive.

Guillermo Acevedo, my creative technology director for the past decade, is the first person I consult with on all matters related to technology. In 2018, Mariluz Hoyos, Madeline Ludwig-Leone, and I launched an art salon where we supported creators in making risk-taking new work. I collaborated with graphic and fashion design friends Xing-Zhen Chung-Hilyard and Melissa Kirgan on several seasons of their fashion line Eko-

Lab, and I invited them to design the costume and headdress for my installation opera *Paradise Interrupted*, 2015. For architectural or structural questions, the first person I contact is Matthew Hilyard, who also contributed to the stage design of *Paradise Interrupted*.

During the pandemic I partnered with Nyssa Chow on a project, and it shook my world. Daniel Arturo Almeida first came to me as a studio assistant. Now the three of us have an ongoing oral history collaboration. I met Charlotte Cohen in 1999 while assisting on a New York City Percent for Art project. Now that I am embarking on my own Percent for Art commission, I continue to call on Charlotte, who heads the Association for Public Art in Philadelphia, for advice and consultation. These amazing individuals, among many others, are not only collaborators and colleagues, but also a part of my chosen family.

Young artists often ask me, what if people don't give back and I get taken advantage of? The answer is straightforward; you don't have to invite them twice when there is no reciprocation. You can't build with people who don't contribute, but if you are willing to take the risk to initiate, in time you'll be surrounded by kindred spirits.

I have intentionally built a multi-generational community, so wisdoms, perspectives, and support could flow in various directions. Fostering such a community takes constant care and upkeep. Finding balance between maintaining a solitary studio practice and spending time with nourishing people is key to longevity, happiness, and artistic well-being.

## SLOW AND STEADY

I've not had gallery representation in my career thus far. I've maintained positive relationships with galleries in the past and continue to partner with them on a project-to-project basis. Given the large scale and ephemeral nature of my practice, museums and public/private institutions are more natural partners through commissioned projects.

A budget for a commission would include an artist fee to compensate for my creative work, in addition to covering project expenses. Due to the lack of standards in the art world, these fees vary widely, often barely covering my studio's overhead and rarely sustaining a livelihood. Consequently, I need to find collectors to acquire artworks as a means of making a living. Aside from securing revenue, I try to keep the studio operating expenses low, which is a challenging task, given my affinity to making large-scale, multi-disciplinary projects, and collaborating with artists, designers, technologists, and others. I also love doing research as an integral part of the creative process, sometimes spanning years of exploration and learning before an artwork or series materializes.

My practice is characterized by a deliberate and measured approach rooted in a lifelong commitment. While urgency in realizing an idea exists, I am not panicked when resources are not immediately available. I always have multiple ongoing concepts, themes, and series under development simultaneously. Collaborating with curators from an inviting institution, I can identify the right project at the right scale and budget.

This practice has taken years to build and is an evolving process. The COVID-19 pandemic has significantly impacted the artworld. I turned 50 last year. I am readjusting to the new external and internal landscapes of the artworld and my own being.

Thinking about and making art in the studio are the most soul-quenching activities I do, despite the uncertainty and anxiety this life brings. Deep down I am at peace to follow this path. I might get lost in the wilderness at times, I might meet a bear that wants to maul me, but I'm right in this world. Slow and steady wins the race.

## BOSSES

I've held many jobs to support my living and artmaking. The most rewarding experience was working for another artist. The years I spent in Cai Guo-Qiang's studio, from 1999 to 2006, were formative in my development. Cai's conceptual breath, daring nature, attention to detail, and ability to amass and command a team to realize a vision have continued to inspire me.

In my own studio, I make it a point to hire young artists, as assistants, project managers, researchers, interns, full time, part time, long term, or in short stints. I keep my practice transparent, so while they contribute to my career, I hope they are learning too—not only from what I do well, but also from my mistakes. I always believed that knowing what you don't want is as important as knowing what you do want!

My life and work have been incredibly enriched by all the young people who have flowed through my studio. I love learning from them and it's a joy to see them thrive after our working relationships end and we forge new ones together.

## ART IS A PROFESSION

This statement used to make me uncomfortable. I wasn't good at asking to be treated as a professional for the work I did out of passion and love. It took me time to learn the skills to demand proper treatment, compensation, and respect for my creative output. I first needed to recognize that the years of education and training to become an artist, dedication, and seriousness at the practice of making good art, and constant time and energy invested in improving and reinventing oneself were worthy of these demands. I believe in artists' power and necessity to society, evident by the innate drive to create art to express the human condition.

Large-scale projects involve working with and managing people. It is important to me that each team member is treated professionally, equitably, and given agency in our collaboration, no matter what role each of us holds. I want the artistic mission to bind us in creating the best work possible, utilizing each of our unique skillsets, perspectives, and experiences.

Working with a professional coach for nearly a decade has fortified my artistic practice by making the above statements a reality. My coach, Charlene Birk, who has also been my best friend since college, assists me with self-leadership by helping setting objectives, holding me accountable for the hard work required to achieve them, providing tools and data to make better decisions, and cheering me on when I achieve goals, whether large or small. Charlene also reminds me that my path is my own, not to be compared to the achievements of others, and encourages me to focus on where I come from and where I need to go, and to take time to appreciate the present moment that I am in.

## ART IS LIFE

Beyond what I have shared, I've also had cats, therapists, and lovers on my journey. I blissfully have a partner who gets me. I need to make love regularly, not just sexual physical love, but also in mind and spirit, with beautiful soulful energies in this world. It is all a part of the alchemistic procreation process of making art. ●

# JOHN SABRAW

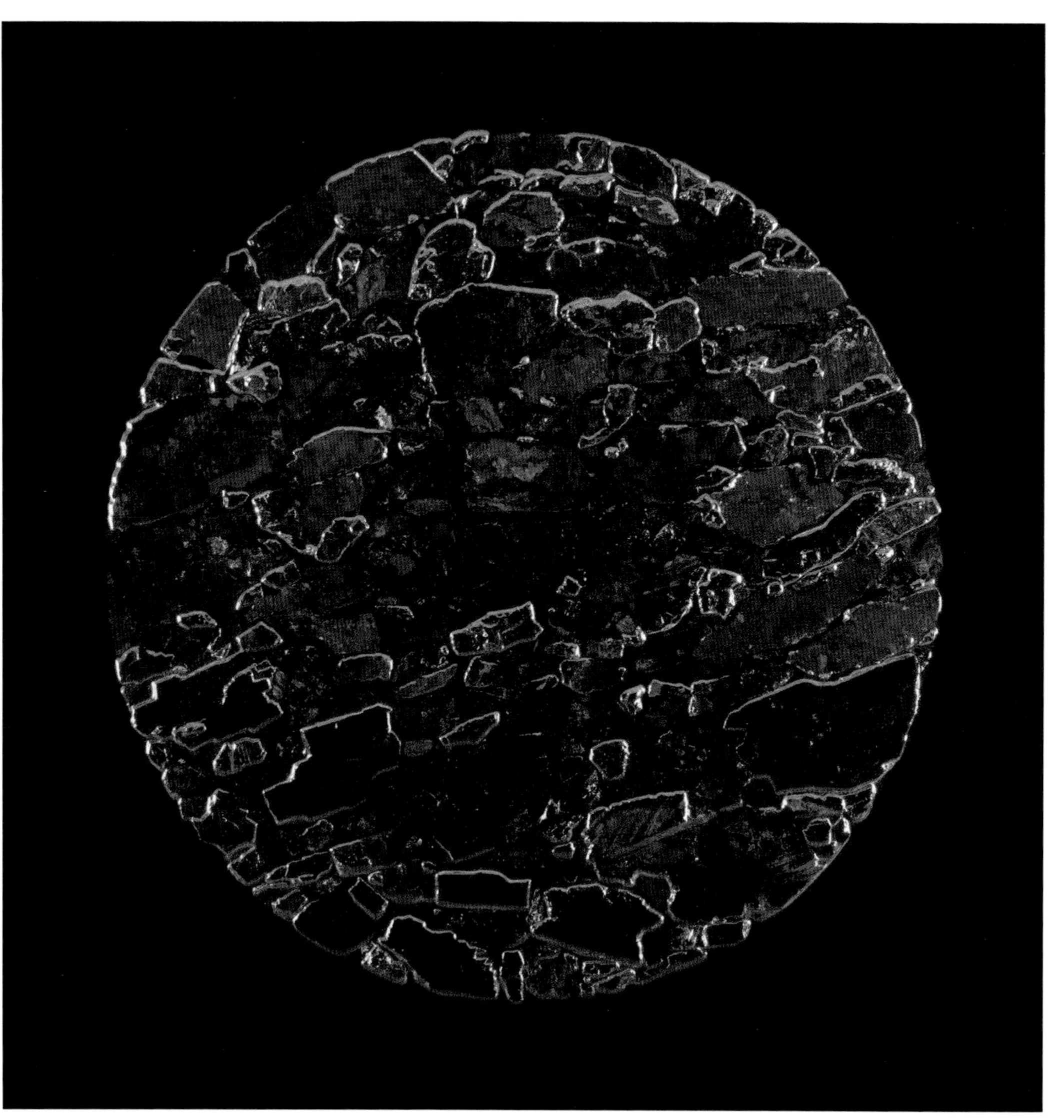

"I WOULD BE ashamed of myself if I was John"—read the note; it wasn't wrong. I was failing nearly every class in high school, including art. College was not in the conversation. But one day while I was skipping school, my art teacher, Pat Nemchock, took my art out of the trashcan (where I had tossed it) and had it reviewed by Congressional Art Competition jurors. I won for the state of Kansas. I was shocked.

Pat helped me put slides together and apply to art schools. I got a partial scholarship to Pratt Institute. I wanted to be an illustrator because it was the only thing I knew you could do creatively. In the summer of 1986 I headed to Brooklyn, New York.

Everyone else seemed to know what art school was all about. I had no clue. I'd never even been to a city; zero street smarts; a rube. I was in a new two-year program for an associate's degree because I could not afford to pursue a four-year program. I lived on the main campus in Brooklyn, but I commuted to Manhattan every day as the program was in the Puck building on Houston Street. One day I was jumped on the subway.

I was really angry after that. So I joined the Guardian Angels, perhaps with some notion of fighting back. I met the first two crew members, one was named Shogun—a martial artist—the other guy I called Mountain, for obvious reasons. They peeled back the complexities of the city as I rode the trains with our

John Sabraw
*Black Mirror*
2021
48″x48″
Coal, coal dust, acrylic resin on honeycomb aluminum panel
Courtesy of the artist

crew of four. Gradually I realized that the crew was aware that a 120-pound white boy was probably going to be the first casualty in any situation, so we were just doing safe train runs and I realized that I was holding back the mission.

In 1987, during my second year at Pratt, Peter Jackson, an editor at Orchard Books, visited as a guest speaker. He showed us how to create a children's book: make a dummy, write a manuscript, etc. I dropped mine off and Peter called me the next day and gave me a contract to write and illustrate it.

Thanks to great camaraderie from my friends Wayne, Roger, Shelley, Michelle, and so many more, in the spring of 1988 I graduated from Pratt with an associate's degree in illustration and I moved into an apartment in nearby Greenpoint, Brooklyn, with my buddy Chris. I spent the summer of 1988 rewriting and illustrating my children's book *I Wouldn't Be Scared*, living off the meager advance. This is what I thought was going to be my life: a children's book illustrator and author.

In 1989 my book was finally printed and Peter had me do some gigs at bookstores and schools promoting the book. I was filled with anxiety each time because I questioned myself: "what does a 20-year-old know about anything?" One time I did a talk with students at an elementary school, but instead of talking with just one class of students, much to my surprise, the entire school attended: children in Kindergarten through sixth grade! I didn't know what to do, so I had the teachers bring out a big pad of paper and a bunch of markers. I ran through the audience asking the kids to describe aspects of characters they might put into a children's book. Then I would run up to the stage and draw the characters they described with the marker as a cartoon, which kind of made a collective children's book together on the fly. I must have lost five pounds in nervous sweat alone—I thought no one was ever going to invite me to anything after that disaster.

Then I got a box in the mail that had dozens of handmade letters from those same kids. Some had drawn their own children's books, and they wrote things like "I am going to be an author when I grow up." I had never had anything so life-affirming as this box of letters. That was the first time I realized that sharing my creative impulses with other people might be of value. And the inkling that maybe teaching was in my future.

None of my other manuscripts of children's books were picked up through 1989, and the royalties from my only book were scant and disappearing. I had to find a job. I answered an ad in the *Village Voice* for a sketcher and got an interview. They took me to a conference room, put a purse on the table in front of me, gave me a blue ballpoint pen and a piece of xerox paper, and said "draw the purse" and left. They came back in, looked at my drawing, and said "you're hired." Suddenly I had a job at a handbag company, Bagland, on 33rd Street and 5th Avenue in Manhattan.

There were three of us "creatives" working at the handbag company: me, Gwen Byrne, and Barbara Lehman. We each had our own drawing table right next to each other shoved into a corner because no one wanted to deal with us. We would do drawings of all of the bags and styles so the sales people could show clients.

I didn't know anything about handbags. I left that job because one of our clients asked for some accessory handbag designs. One of them was a cigarette case, which I drew up as a coffin. Jobless, I tried to be a freelance illustrator, but I never did what the editors wanted me to do so that work dried up. At one point, I even went out to Minneapolis, Minnesota, and tried to be an advertising person for two weeks.

I returned to New York and got a job working at William Doyle auction house on 87th Street cleaning and setting up incoming furniture. My boss was Patrick Ameche, who acted in some Andy Warhol films. Patrick and I were in the tag sale division, which retailed items that weren't auction quality—mostly to antique dealers, a hilariously entertaining and competitive group. It was a strange place with interesting people and celebrities popping in like Michael Douglas, Audrey Meadows, Catherine Deneuve, etc. But it was still just a temporary, non-sustainable gig.

With the children's author path dead, I now thought I was going to be the next "Spike Lee" as a film director. I bought an 8-millimeter camera and wrote terrible scripts, trying to convince my friends to act in them. In 1990, I was accepted to the Vancouver Film Institute. But I needed money to attend. One day at work I was cleaning out a chest of drawers that came in, and I found a set of rings. They were comical, like from a vending machine—plastic rings with giant gemstones. I thought it would be hilarious to give these to my girlfriend. Patrick was like "sure just let me just clear it next door." Turns out the rings were very real, antique, and worth thousands of dollars. I asked the owner if he would give me enough money to go to film school since I had found these rings and turned them in: nope. I would not be going to film school after all—and I would also not be employed there anymore.

I was crushed, even more lost and really needed a J-O-B. I was hired by another handbag company, Mitzi, right across the street from the old one where I previously worked. I was given an American Express credit card and would buy thousands of dollars' worth of luxury handbags, bring them back to the office and make designs that were similar. Then I'd return the bags to each store where they were purchased. I was sent to the Dominican Republic where I trained factory workers to create the handbags. I was sent to design houses in Taipei and Hong Kong. It was an incredible experience to have only at the age of 21. I became enamored with a big world. The self-doubt and all of those things—they were all still there—but now I had been energized to build a life.

Cara, one of my coworkers at Mitzi, pulled me aside when I came back from Hong Kong and informed me (through my jetlagged brain) that our other coworker Carmen had a romantic interest in me. Cara then dragged me to a party in New Jersey, where Carmen was there. At the end of the party I offered to chaperone Carmen on her late-night train trek all the way to her apartment in Astoria, Queens. Once there she dismissed me, and in my dead-tired travel fog I told her what Cara said. Carmen was shocked as she had no interest in me. So we made a plan to prank Cara back. We went on a fake movie date, prepared to then tell lavish stories of how bad it was to make Cara regret making this up. We've now been married 32 years.

A few months into the gig, I was home to visit family and visited a group exhibition of work by the faculty at the University of Kansas (KU). I saw a painting by Robert Brawley, and I had never seen a work of art by a living human who could paint this way. I reached out and talked with him. It's the first time in a long time that I felt that I had a pull in some kind of direction that felt right; maybe I was supposed to be an artist, a painter . . . I wanted to study painting in New York City, but couldn't afford it. I did not want to study in Kansas, yet it was so cheap to go to school at KU because the cost of living was a fraction of what it was compared to NYC, and Robert was there. In July 1991, I made the decision to move back to Kansas and study painting at the University of Kansas.

I bought a used '76 Chevy Caprice Classic car and lived out of it for 40 days and 40 nights, seeing 11,000 miles of the American West with my friend Dan Bailey. After that trip, I moved to Lawrence, Kansas, and got a job assembling explosives for helicopter hooks. Carmen joined me there, and we got married in 1992.

In 1993, I was accepted into the BFA Painting program at KU. It was very difficult coming from an illustration background to learn fine arts, and I am so grateful to my friends in the program for helping me through this: Megan, Scott, Ed, James, Betsy, Shawna, and so many more. I knew this was what I wanted to do. As I was finishing my BFA in 1994, Robert Brawley curated a show with Mongerson Wunderlich, his gallery in Chicago, at the Art Expo Chicago Navy Pier and included my work in it! My three little paintings sold during that exhibition and Mongerson began showing my work.

That summer Carmen and I packed up our belongings in Kansas and moved to Chicago. I got a job working at the Goods of Evanston arts supply store in Evanston, Illinois, a suburb of Chicago. I applied to Northwestern University's MFA program to study with artist James Valerio. While working at Goods of Evanston, artist Robert Gamblin was personally repping his own paint, Gamblin Artist Colors. He would come in and share his paint and teach us different ways of using it.

In 1995 I was accepted into the Northwestern University (NU) MFA program with a fellowship. I felt like I had won the lottery. The Union League Club in Chicago has a scholarship program for the arts, and in the last year of my studies at NU, I was awarded a Union League Club scholarship and the juror for that year was Chicago gallery dealer Tom McCormick. Later, Tom came to my MFA thesis show in 1997 and offered me a solo exhibition in his gallery the next year.

Right at that time, my daughter Isa was born, so I needed to make money fast! Thanks to a tip from artist Anna Kunz I was able to get a job working for the American Academy of Art in Chicago, not teaching, but recruiting and doing administrative work. Each week, my schedule was working sixteen hour days for four days in a row. The commute to work was an hour each way, each day, and then I had a three-day weekend to supposedly paint in the studio. But our baby was a handful. I was barely in my studio. A couple months before the show scheduled with Tom McCormick, I had to tell him that I would not have enough work to do the solo show. I was feeling bleak. Carmen and I realized we could not afford to live on the meager salary I was earning. We decided we needed to have a major change in expenses for a short period of time so we could reset. We looked into moving to a small town outside Chicago or outside of New York, but could not afford it. So we asked to spend a few months in my mother's home back in Kansas—it was our last option.

On advice from Anna, I wrote Tom a letter apologizing, explaining that we were moving away, that I was going to try to make art when I could, and if I made anything good I'd reach out. I felt like shit. I knew I was going to find a job and responsibly provide for our family, but I also felt that this was the death of my art career.

Tom got the letter and called me and asked if I had any art done at all. I told him I had a few paintings that were halfway done. He and his wife Janice wanted to come by the studio and see what I was working on. Embarrassed, I said don't bother. But he insisted. They came to the studio and offered me a solo show for the next year (I am sure Anna had a hand in this). Stunned, I accepted. I told Carmen what happened and she said she would take care of Isa, live with us in her mother-in-law's house, and support me any way she could, making art full time for the exhibit at Tom's for one year to try to spark my gallery success and land a teaching gig. At the end of the year, if art sales and/or teaching art weren't enough to fund us living independently, I had to do whatever it took to provide for the family. I agreed.

In 1998 in Kansas I was on a fucking mission. I swore I would not disappoint anyone ever again. In Lawrence, I rented the windowless cinder block storage space at the back of a portrait studio in a strip mall for $150 a month. That year was absolute hell, but I made 22 paintings and I had my solo show in the winter of 1999 at Tom's. We sold about half the show, and I got a review in the *Chicago Reader* by Fred Camper, and in The New Art Examiner by Diane Thodos. Meanwhile I was in my third year of applying for teaching jobs with over 100 "thank you, but no" letters already, but I had two first round interviews that winter.

Months passed. The few thousand dollars I made from those art sales in Chicago didn't begin to cover our credit card debt. My year of art was done. As promised, in spring 1999 I got a job—answering a help line for the federal financial aid office. After a month, I got invited for an on-campus interview at Washington University in St. Louis as a one-year lecturer in foundations position. A few weeks later I had my first full-time teaching job.

We moved to St. Louis and I was so grateful to have a position teaching. Unfortunately, for my first couple of years, I tried to pound a lifetime of teaching into every single student. I overwhelmed everyone, but it was an invigorating and rewarding atmosphere. I met St. Louis gallerist Elliot Smith at one of his openings and a bit later showed him my work. He put a few of my paintings in a group show in 2001 and they sold. This led to a small solo show later that year. After that we sold several paintings a year for the next few years, which allowed my art practice to break even, which meant that my small salary from Wash U almost covered living expenses.

Post 9/11, I began teaching art and activism courses. I wrote a letter to the newspaper in protest of the impending second invasion of Iraq and someone doxed me: my mailman brought boxes of hate mail some of which said things like, "You're Satan," "you don't have Jesus in your heart," and "you're not a patriot," and threats of violence. I felt I had put my family in harm's way—it was terrifying. I realized that yelling into the void wasn't getting me anywhere. I began to ask myself, "what was I, as a father, doing to build a future that I wanted my daughter to be in? What was I doing as a professor to encourage students' voices? What was my art practice in light of these things as well?" I realized that the war, colonial legacy, and so many other things I was concerned with were factors of inequality, and inequality was about power and exploitation of resources: e.g., sustainability and climate justice. I didn't know much yet, but I felt I could have an impact in these areas and try to build a future that my students and my daughter could live in, enjoy, and be proud of.

In 2003, my daughter was old enough to start school, but we could not find anything affordable or acceptable in St. Louis, so I began looking for new teaching positions. I had a couple of offers, one of them at Ohio University. When I visited the local elementary school in the neighborhood where I thought we wanted to live, the class of kindergartners were of mixed race like my daughter, mixed religions, etc., which made me feel it was the right move. Athens, Ohio, is a very small town, so it was a big shift, but our daughter was able to walk to school by herself and roam the neighborhoods and woods with friends.

Continuing my push into sustainability and climate justice, in 2009 I started teaching an experimental course titled "Save the World." The premise of the course was for all of the students to figure out how they would save the world in one semester, only to realize it's impossible. From that realization, they worked in small groups, and they would filter down to a demographic that they felt they could have an impact on. The final exam was that they had to execute an activist artwork in public.

While teaching those classes my students were like "you're making us do this, but what are you doing?" Good question. I started looking at my own practice. That's the first time I questioned where am I getting my paints from? Where am I getting my lumber from? My water, my electricity, my gas, and everything else?

Working with carbonfund.org in 2009, I created an algorithm that had a web-based interface where artists could go and put in how many artworks they made in a year, and it would calculate for them their carbon footprint and give them a link where they could go and buy carbon credits to offset their greenhouse emissions. It was clunky, but an important step for me because about this time a group of environmental faculty introduced me to acid mine drainage. It's pollution from abandoned coal mines that kills over 1,300 miles of streams in Ohio alone. The streams smell of sulfur and are this vibrant orange color—which is iron oxide sludge. My first thought was, "can I make paint out of this stuff?" I took a jar of sludge back to my studio and made completely unusable paint. A few months later a friend asked if I would meet with her professor, Guy Riefler, who needed an artists' help.

Riefler, it turns out, had the same idea! We started asking what if the iron sludge could be sold as a valuable pigment rather than disposed of as a waste product? What if treating pollution could be an entrepreneurial endeavor rather than a societal cost? For many years though, we could not get significant funding or buy into our idea. We really needed an industry partner that could prove our pigments to be marketable. I hoped that working with Robert Gamblin all those years ago could be an ice breaker, and it was. Once Gamblin Artists Colors tested our pigments for safety and quality, they made 500 tubes of oil paint. Through a Kickstarter campaign in 2018 these paints were distributed to artists around the world.

I write this in early 2024, we have just completed ground preparation for our full-scale treatment facility in Truetown, Ohio, that will restore the next seven miles of Sunday creek, create a habitat for aquatic life, treat over one million gallons of acid mine drainage pollution and produce over 6,000 pounds of sustainably sourced iron oxide pigment, every day for the next several generations. The sale of this pigment will pay for plant operations, jobs, and profits will go to clean up more streams.

The ice caps are melting, the air is unbreathable, and there is not enough water. There are astounding species that are dying off, and war and famine—it's all just incredibly dark and depressing. But the thing that I have learned through all of the years I have been doing this is that when people come from very different backgrounds to creatively work on a problem together, it is joyous and life affirming and often successful.

I love painting in my hermetic studio bubble. Yet, being able to utilize my creativity in meetings with engineers deciding on wetland design, or building compelling visual presentations to gain entrepreneurial funding, or supporting the ideas and ideals of many people who want to have some positive impacts, are an equal part of my creative life. It is the exploration of how my creative self can contribute and thrive in all these different roles and the inspirational people I get to meet in the process that has made my life so rich and fulfilling. •

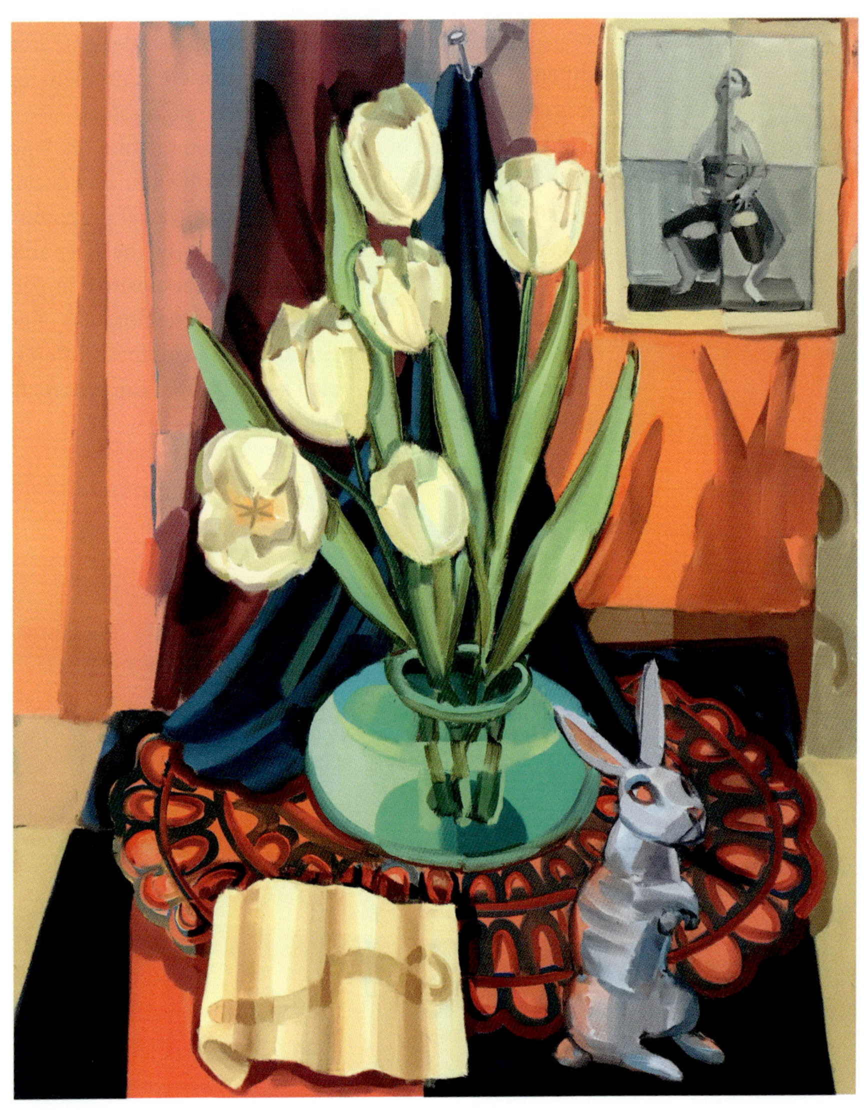

I WAS BORN to an 18-year-old mother in 1940 in Pasadena, California with no resources in a pre-prosperity America. She survived, and prospered, and was able to assist me in important ways. I was an only child raised in different landscapes in and around Los Angeles, from the high desert Newhall, East LA, to the beach cities of Hermosa and Manhattan Beach.

In 1958, I attended the California College of Arts and Crafts in Oakland, California. My parents paid my tuition and I also worked as a nanny, a dishwasher, and afterschool recreation instructor. I met and married Philip Linhares and gave birth to my daughter shortly after my 20th birthday in my second year of art school. After a six-month break, I resumed my commitment to getting my degree. My young husband (and fellow art student) worked as a florist and continued his education, while my parents gave us $200 a month. I was awarded a scholarship every year going forward and received my undergraduate degree in five years. My parents wanted me to get a degree in education. Like all parents they were eager to see me become financially independent. Their vision for me was to be a high school art teacher and have summers off to go the beach. I had bigger dreams.

In the early 1960s, Oakland had a city-sponsored childcare facility where parents paid according to their income for childcare. This was an amazing program, and a terrific help. I

Judith Linhares
*Go Tell Alice*
2022
35 1/2″x26″
Oil on linen
Courtesy of the artist and
P·P·O·W Gallery, New York

also had two girlfriends I relied on to exchange babysitting. This was really important and helped me in my effort to continue to develop as an artist.

In 1963, I left my husband and started graduate school at the California College of Arts and Crafts. My parents continued to send me small amounts of money. While I attended graduate school, I worked at the childcare center where my daughter was attending. This was a full-time job. Later I worked as a substitute teacher in Oakland Public schools. All the while I was keeping in contact with other serious-minded artists and finding time and space to work. Graduate school provided a built-in community of artists with whom I shared ideas and attended museum and gallery shows. The Bay Area had a lively bohemian art scene. Peter Voulkos, the ceramic master, was teaching at the University at Berkeley. He had a huge warehouse space where he lived and worked and hosted large parties with live music. These parties became a place to meet and collaborate with other artists. I like to keep in mind that it was a very different time; living was cheap. In 1964, I moved from Oakland to San Francisco. The standard of living in California was high; rents for beautiful apartments with windows in every room were plentiful low and finding temporary employment was also easy.

During my graduate school days, I was living in a large flat with room to work, I think the rent was around $60 a month. I continued to work in public schools and various other "interesting" jobs. One wonderful job I had was making art projects with children in public parks, which was very fun, and I had no supervision so even better.

I met my next romantic partner in 1964 and moved with him into a warehouse in San Francisco. We showered at the San Francisco Art Institute, which was a short drive from the loft where we lived. I was still substitute teaching. My parents no longer were giving me funds. I began to meet many other artists and we hosted drawing sessions in our apartment. We moved again in 1965 near the Haight Ashbury district where young people were coming in droves from all over the country. We went to many marches for civil rights, protests against the war, and rock concerts. It was part of a time that belonged to the young.

I continued to develop my work. I used the living room in the apartment for my studio. I worked for about a year at a recreation center for the physically challenged. This too was an interesting job with quite a bit of responsibility. I quit after about a year as I felt I was not a professional social worker—I was not a trained art therapist and needed to concentrate on my art.

As a result of developing my work and artist-to-artist connections, I applied for and received a college teaching job in 1966 at a new school in downtown San Francisco. This school became the San Francisco Art Academy. This position, along with the substitute teaching, sharing expenses with my partner, and renting out a spare room in our flat, got me through the next couple of years.

I had always considered myself a feminist, so when the second wave of the feminist movement came along in the 1960s, I was ready. I belonged to a woman's consciousness-raising group. In the Bay Area, I knew all of the women involved before we started meeting. They were all artists whose work I respected. Some of them I had shown with in local galleries. Most of these women were recent graduates from one of the several art schools or university graduate programs. While our art was not similar, all approaches and materials were practiced. We met a couple of times a month. For ten years, we showed together, traveled together, and many of them are still close friends.

At first, the meetings centered around complaining about our boyfriends, then complaining about our mothers. When we were through complaining, the meetings became about art. This context was my first experience of having a studio visit.

The result of looking closely at how women had been discriminated against in hiring practices began to be an issue in institutions in 1969. At the time, I had experience, energy, ideas, and my work. As I recall, I had no women teachers in painting or in graduate school. However, I had some wonderful women teachers in design, weaving, and ceramics. I was the only woman in my class to graduate with an MFA from California College of Arts and Crafts.

After graduation I took a one-year, full-time position teaching at San Jose City College in 1970. I also had my first solo exhibition that year. I called the show *Love Letters from San Jose*. I moved to San Jose, rented a storefront with an apartment and a backyard, and moved in with my then 10-year-old daughter. I exchanged a room for childcare with a local college student. Her schedule allowed her to be at home when my daughter came home from school. I loved my students who were mostly Chicano veterans returning from Vietnam. I taught them and they taught me so much more. Even though this was a wonderful experience, I felt I needed to be in an environment with serious, ambitious fellow artists and access to museums. I will say it was great to be able to buy new underwear, have my car fixed, and pay my bills.

I moved back to San Francisco a single woman again. I rented an apartment in the Noe Valley area of San Francisco. I worked in the living room, my daughter had the bedroom, and I had a bed in the pantry. The place had a terrible roach problem.

Upon my return to San Francisco, I worked many adjunct teaching positions getting by well enough. Selling art was not anything that artists thought about as there wasn't a real commercial art scene in San Francisco. Getting rich off of one's art was not a dream anyone had. I still have all the art from my first show in 1971.

In 1972, my parents put a down payment on a house in San Francisco. I made the payments on the mortgage. The wisdom I received from my parents was that when buying property, it is good to have a source of income so I purchased a two-flat building. I made my studio in the basement, collected rent to pay the mortgage, and lived rent free while teaching in various colleges in the Bay Area.

This situation was good for a while. In 1978, my work was included in an important show in New York called *Bad Painting* at Marcia Tucker's New Museum. I came to New York for the show and stayed for a couple of weeks. It was not love at first sight between New York City and myself.

On my return to San Francisco, I began to think about moving to New York. I had a few friends who had been living in NYC for years. In 1978, I also had a semester visiting artist position at Louisiana State University (LSU) in Baton Rouge. I took it in part because I needed a break from San Francisco. I was restless. My daughter was living her own independent life and my reasons for being in San Francisco were becoming less compelling. The next step for me would be to secure a tenured teaching position in a university. I felt I had too much energy to make settling down my destiny at that particular point.

In 1978, I met a man in Baton Rouge who I would spend the next 36 years with. We lived together in San Francisco for a couple of years and then set out in a large rental truck across the country to New York City. I kept my house in San Francisco and collected rent for a number of years. I have never regretted the move. I like the intense atmosphere and constant conversation with fellow artists in New York. There is a sense that culture is important and everyone is in agreement. It puts wind in my sails. I turned 40 in New York City and I have now lived half of my life here.

The first few years in New York City were hard, but fruitful. In 1980, we secured a rent-stabilized loft in TriBeCa. I had a solo show at Concord Gallery, which was a decent gallery at the time. These were lucky breaks.

I had a built a community of friends I had met in San Francisco. They were very helpful in sharing information about galleries and explaining to me how to work with a gallery, how things were done then. The exhibition came about by showing slides of work to gallery directors to see if they might be interested. The director liked the work and gave me a show. The gallery closed before I could have a second show. Then figuration fell out of favor. I continued to show in group shows but did not have another solo show in New York City for ten years.

I have always had a lot of support from fellow artists and I do not take this for granted; I consider it very important. I have a circle of friends that I talk about art with. They have been key to my confidence and development. I have kept in touch with many of the women that were involved in the women's group from the 1970s, too.

I lived in New York City on a minimal amount of money for many years, surviving because I shared my expenses, had a rent-controlled space, and a not large but basic salary from teaching at the School of Visual Arts and New York University. I was fortunate enough to receive a few generous grants from the National Endowment for the Arts, the John Simon Guggenheim Memorial Foundation, and other foundations. These grants helped me buy time to work and purchase materials. It seemed that whenever my credit card was near its limit, I would receive a grant. This has been quite a tight rope act. I do not believe I could have allowed myself this lifestyle if I did not know that I would at some point inherit some funds. It was never clear if it would be enough to live on, but it did give me the courage to live a more precarious life financially.

In 2012, I did inherit money; I am single again. I am no longer teaching. I quit teaching in 2017. I bought a building in Brooklyn, New York. I have the studio of my dreams. I love Brooklyn. Things are very good for me right now. •

KATINKA MANN

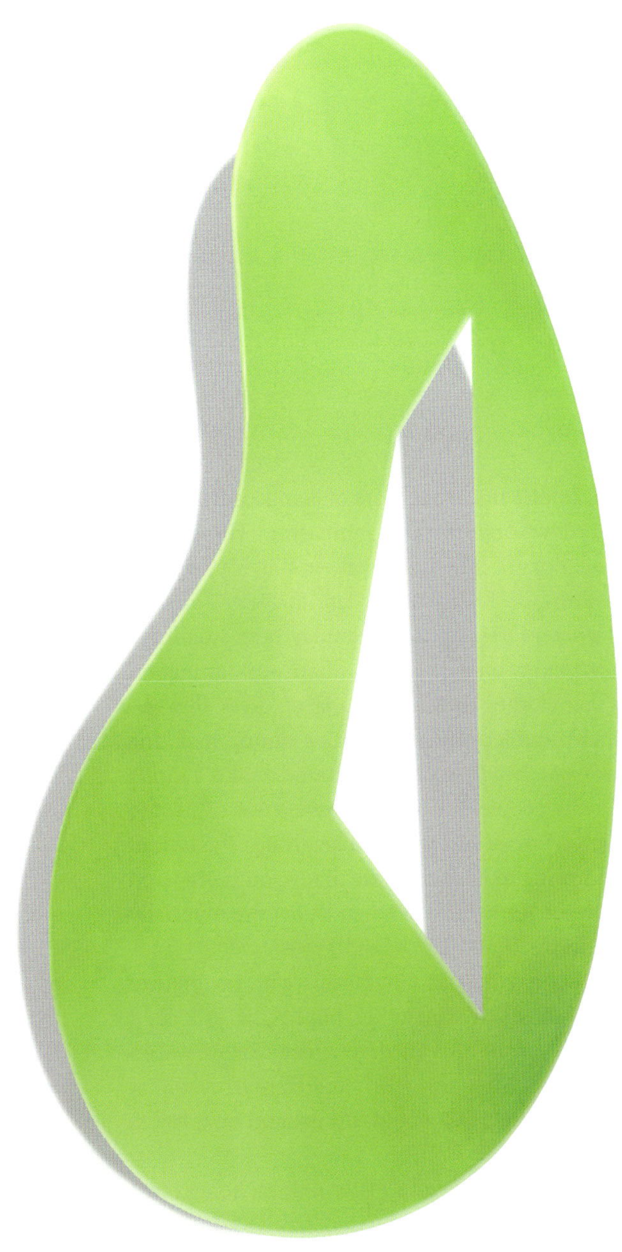

MY POSITIVE attitude came from years of being a survivor.

I was born in New York City to parents from Hungary in 1925. The first memory I can remember was at 6 years old. Walking on a boardwalk, I was somewhere in New York, too young to recall where. Dressed in my Sunday best, holding a man's hand. I didn't know him, or why or where our destination was. I changed my clothes into a set code of dress that the orphanage had and was led into a darkened dining hall. The only lights were from lanterns on each round table. I didn't remember seeing any people. My only awareness was of a witch flying around the perimeter of the room, laughing. The lack of knowing what was going to happen to me in my youth prepared me for a field with the same instability, and I believe especially for women artists in the 1960s, 1970s, and 1980s.

I remember living for one-and-a-half years with my mother and brother. I never lived with my father, but he always looked after me in his special way until he died. As a teenager, we would meet in New York City and go to a Horn and Hardart Automat or other places once a week. We would just eat and talk. It was our time.

At the age of 10, I began living in foster homes, being most fortunate that three of my four extended families in foster homes had a loving atmosphere. I saw love and goodness in relationships through my foster families. In my second and third extended families, we went to the country for the summers. The

Katinka Mann
*The Source*
2021
62″(h)x 37″(w)x1/4″(d)
Painted aluminum, flattened sculptural painting
Courtesy of the Katinka Mann Estate
Photography by Garrett Carroll

women in these families were sisters. The freedom of being in the midst of nature started a love affair that planted seeds of being at one with nature. It was an amazing, silent gift. I had no idea at that time how it would emerge years later and become central to my art and life.

At 15 and-a-half, I moved to my fourth foster parents located in Brooklyn. It took one-and-a-half hours to get to my high school each day. After school, I worked at Woolworths on 5th Avenue in the dish department, in the basement of the store, nineteen hours a week; my pay was $12. Two years of this very full schedule set a pattern for the rigors of working in the 1960s.

I was under the care of the Federation of Jewish Philanthropies of New York until I was 16. Discussions with my social worker stressed how important it was for me to have at least a high school diploma. I was most fortunate. They agreed to support me until 18 years of age. It was an important lesson for me in learning how to keep on my path.

In my fourth foster home, the parents had two daughters. Mimi was the oldest. She developed into a vivacious, creative personality full of energy and love. Whenever the family got together for an occasion, she created a field of warmth and love.

Years later, she wove her charisma into each of her four children as well as leaving her mark on all of us. I am still deeply touched each and every time we are together 79 years later. Mimi's vibration of love helped me to express and care for my own family. She showed me how to bring light and love into my life.

In 1945, when I was 20, I met my future husband Joe, whom I married in 1947. We shared a love of dance and music. We lived in a two-bedroom apartment shared with a co-worker of mine. New York apartments weren't easy to find, after the war. I gave birth to our first daughter in 1950. After a month, my mother came for a visit. We were sitting and I put baby Joan in her arms. She looked down and her first words were, "I can't stand to look at her." Her negativity was so toxic that my insides recoiled. Showing my mother to the door, I told her, "I never wanted to see her again." She strengthened my determination to see the positive side of life.

My first oil painting class was taken in an adult education program. Never having been exposed to art, my first work caused an awakening in me. I believe the universe spurred something within me that needed to continue creating. Landscape painting was such a natural fit, I took to it like a sponge.

Four years later, our second daughter was born, making our family complete.

In 1957, my husband was promoted. Joe worked for a firm that sold furniture and bedding. He was transferred to Hartford, Connecticut. The first two weeks after arriving in Hartford was spent registering our daughters in school and getting settled. Luckily, the school was just a few short blocks from our suburban home. Through my daughters, I met my wonderful neighbors who had large families. Whenever I needed help, they were most giving in including my daughters into their homes to be part of the play-time shared with their own children.

I enrolled in classes at the Hartford Art School, University of Hartford in Connecticut. The classes were stimulating. Meeting friends that were on the same wavelength was a special plus. One day at the library, by chance, a small book of verses on Taoism by Lao Tzu called *The Way of Life* came across my path. On my night-table next to my bed was a pad and pencil to catch drawings from dream images and Lao Tzu's book of 81 verses. Each night before turning out the light, I would read one verse. Through its uniting of polarities, it reinforced my sense of wholeness. I was struck by its spiritual luminosity whereby I could join art and life and treat them as one.

Four years later, Joe was promoted, taking us back to New York.

In the 1960s and 1970s, the human potential movement was very strong. Combined with years of attending yoga and meditation at Kripalu in Lenox, Massachusetts, studying Abraham Maslow, workshops with Deepak Chopra, Wayne Dyer, and Jean Houston made me thirsty for new beginnings. Journaling with Jungian psychologist Dr. Ira Progoff and therapy, my feelings opened. I began to understand the hardships my mother must have undergone and forgave her for deserting me.

Our daughters Joan and Amy broadened my field of love and growth. Each stage was a learning experience for all of us.

There were successes and challenges. My daughters gave me the strength to sever my relationship with my mother. I did not want them to be exposed to her negativity. My mother was a remarkable woman for her time. I owe her no blame. She did things to survive in the only way she knew. She made me appreciate a loving relationship with my husband and daughters. She helped me choose the world of being positive. Her gift to me was to be a survivor, which turned out to be a great rescuer in my later years.

In 1961 we bought our house, leaving most of the property as woods so that our family could see the transformation and changing scene of each new season. We had no curtains, only some sliding stained glass windows and a few shutters. Witnessing the cycles of birth and death each year, increased my sense of awe and wonder. Taoism is based on the rhythms of nature.

Living in suburbia in 1966, my thoughts turned to how I could earn extra money. I was having exhibitions, but it wasn't enough monetarily. Loving to teach was very rewarding but financially it wasn't enough. I asked myself, "What service could I offer people that they would want and don't have?" Living an hour from New York City, I missed visiting museums and galleries. My daughters were in school and came home by 3:00 p.m. I wanted to develop a plan which had to revolve around school schedules, geared for mothers like myself. In placing an ad in the free local *Penny Saver*, I founded and directed an art touring business that lasted 25 years. Taking classes in public speaking made addressing groups easier. Researching artists' lives and their work was fascinating. Mostly women attended; about 48 per tour. We played short games to develop our awareness and perceptions. Later listening to each other's art responses and learning from each other was an incredible experience of discovery as well as great fun.

Raising our family, cooking, cleaning, shopping, researching for the art tours, working four days with four different groups from 10:00 a.m. to 2:30 p.m. bi-monthly, working toward an exhibition with new work with a timeline of every two years, time for exploring future new ideas for growth, being a girl scout leader for seven years. I loved everything I was involved with and grew in all the different facets of my endeavors. After my daughters were asleep, I'd go to the studio eager to explore. My husband worked ten hours a day. He fully supported all my involvements. I felt very appreciative in being able to do all the things I loved to do.

Years flew bye, my daughters left home to start their own journeys. Joe had started his own business in bedding and furniture. I concentrated on my art and "Gallery Hopping" tours in the fall and spring. One winter I went on tours in Mexico. Included in the tour were the Pyramids of the Sun and the Moon. The experience blew me away. The next tour we visited four colonial towns including San Miguel. For fourteen years, spending three months of each year in San Miguel De Allende, Mexico, I took classes and had a place to work at the Bellas Artes. Joe was there six weeks each year. We visited different archaeological sites each year. Studying the architecture of prehistoric buildings was compelling. The experiences added to the stimulus developing my first exhibition of shaped abstract reliefs. My work naturally adapted through generational shifts. I'm still expressing in 2020 the same basic premise as I did in the 1960s.

In the 1970s. I was keeping an eye on the exhibitions at a particular gallery on Madison Avenue in New York City (whose name I cannot remember). Feeling my work would fit in with the gallery's direction, I brought my work in to show the owner. She looked through my portfolio. Her kind response was, "No matter how good your work is, I cannot feature a woman artist. Nobody would buy it."

1976 added to my learning curve. I was the sixth member voted into Central Hall Gallery, a women's cooperative gallery in Port Washington, Long Island. We renovated a black oiled two-story high garage into a white gallery space. Having panel discussions, speakers and artist talks, the membership grew beyond the original thirteen. I was a member until its demise in 1983 in New York City. The camaraderie excelled.

With our children gone from the nest, our home started to become a physical and financial burden. The realistic option was to downsize. I was going to miss the woods, but giving up my studio was the hardest. I began the arduous task of giving supplies away. My 24 × 36 inches dry mounting press and an incredible amount of supplies were donated to L. I. University at C. W. Post Art Department in Long Island. Thirty-seven plexiglass boxes were donated to the Huntington Historical Society and the Art League of L. I. Gallery. There were many small works. I called friends offering them to take any one they liked. All the large, shaped paintings were donated to Mimi's sons for their new headquarters. We finally closed on our house, arriving in New York City in January 2006. After an eighteen year wait list, we moved into our four-room apartment in Chelsea, Manhattan. I was lost without a studio.

I found myself in the midst of the biggest battle of my life—for my life. August 2006 was my first surgery for melanoma. After my fourth surgery with melanoma in February 2007, a new decision had to be made. My status was Stage 4, with metastatic, malignant melanoma. Two strong assets were in my past: art and my survivor's instinct that guided me. When an art period had been fully explored, it was time to explore new directions. It seemed the same scenario was happening with melanoma. I changed to an alternative doctor who completely altered my lifestyle. My survival instincts became alive. I took an active role in visualizations. I would imagine the melanoma being washed away. I felt it leaving my body. I meditated, journaled, and listened to chanting on tapes. I would do exercises with white healing light. I made up games creating real wars in my mind's eye, between my red blood cells and white cells, having the right cells win. Meditating in nature and the power of the cosmic force were a strong hold over me. I wanted to live my life just the way it was, loving my family and my involvement in art. Counting my blessings every day, I worked the protocol religiously, just as if working on my art. It worked. In 2007, I had three months to live; I am thirteen years in remission.

In 2007, I applied to the Marie Walsh Sharpe Art Foundation, The Space Program, for a studio. When receiving the incredible news of my selection, I was deeply grateful. Words cannot say enough because it brought my life back to normal. After having a studio at the Marie Walsh Sharpe studio between 2008–09, I was accepted to the Elizabeth Foundation for the Arts studio program in 2009, where my studio is one among a larger community of artists. It doesn't get any better. I have had a studio there ever since.

I find keeping the intention of working paramount. If I'm tired from lack of sleep or whatever the reason, I still go to the studio. It doesn't seem long when I'm alerted to seeing a prospect I didn't see before and the energy starts to buzz. Having the intention of working, makes my practice work. It's putting myself where the action is, which in turn sharpens my instincts among the surrounding stimuli of artists and our community.

My husband Joe was the most important and influential person in my life. In everything that I wanted to do, he supported me 100 percent. When I was faced with difficult decisions, he'd help me see it through. When I had opportunities, he was the first to encourage me to go for it. Our loving and caring daughters and their families (which include four grandchildren and three great grandchildren) and the loving extended family of Mimi's, getting bigger and bigger, are all very special and dear to my heart, as they were to Joe.

When a work was sold, I generally had to install it at that time. It was a given that Joe would do it. He did so many things with a great attitude, happy to be part of the event. When I had melanoma, there were a multitude of physical things that had to be done. Joe never complained, always doing his utmost to help. His greatest gift to me was always encouraging me to pursue my art. When he retired at 89, the last six years of his life, he was the assistant in the studio. He traveled all over the city, to have things made, get estimates, do installations, preparing the final touches for the work to be hung, purchasing art supplies, etc. I felt truly blessed, privileged, and loved. We were married for 70 years.

I am grateful that my art continues to flourish. That there will be many more years of learning and growing, in a state of unending becoming. With the universe as my creative partner, I am in awe of it always teaching me in unexpected ways how to be sensitive to art and life's calling. •

# KAY MILLER

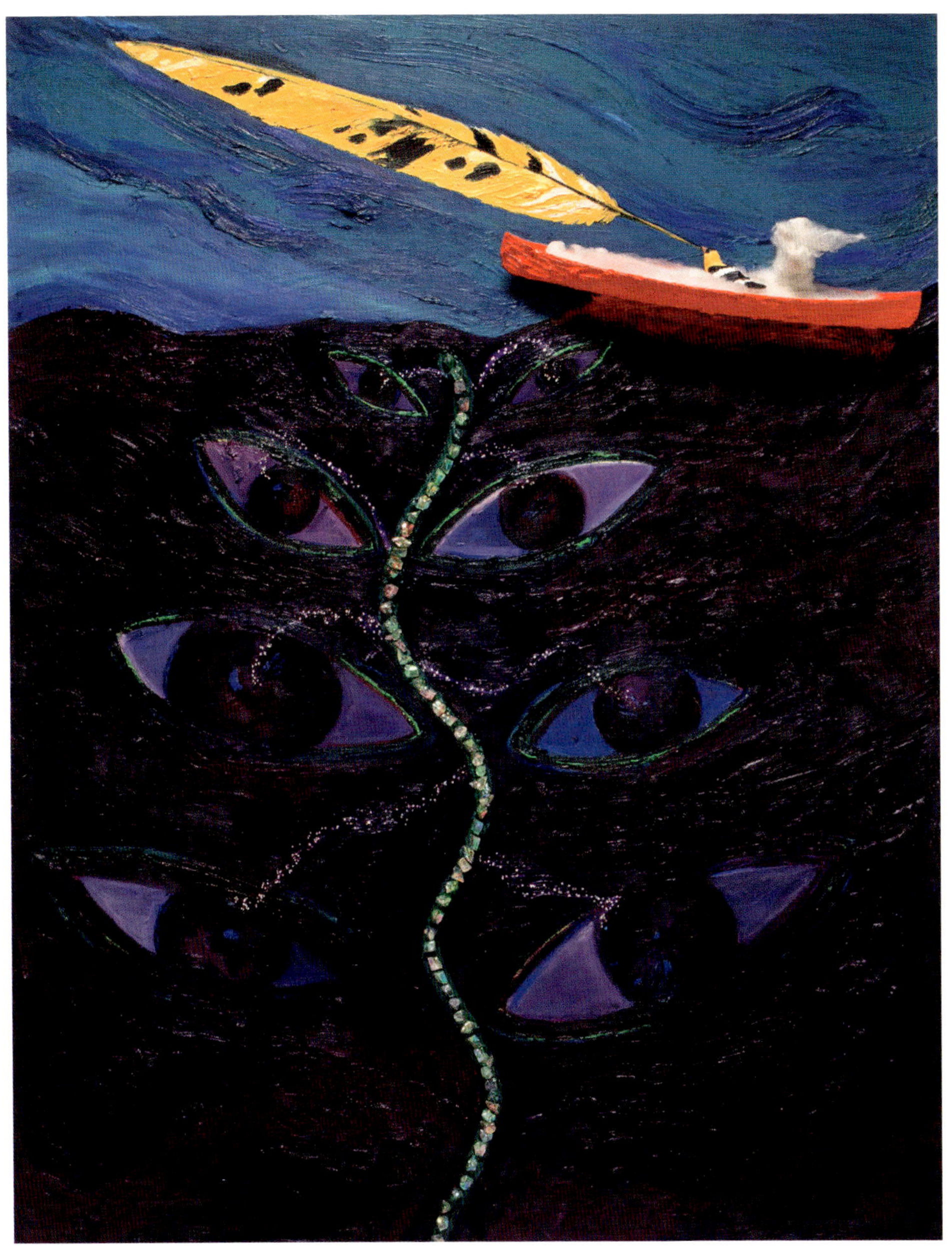

MY MOTHER had an elementary school education; my father had less. They met picking cotton for a landowner in Hillsboro, Texas. Both were highly intelligent, brave, and kind; down-to-earth people of high degree. To sustain a growing family, they left the fields in 1941 for Houston, settling near the ship channel. They were socially isolated and disenfranchised with a displaced culture and lost genealogy. My mother took in laundry, which she hand-washed, line-dried, and ironed. My father unloaded ships and painted houses. He enjoyed color mixing and was a meticulous craftsman, yet his earnings were never more than minimum wage. They suffered the indignities of poverty their entire lives.

We lived in a small house near the Wayside and Navigation intersection known in the mid-1960s as Houston's murder corner. Ironically, my parents were pacifists. Not churchgoers, but they were spiritually tied to nature and were aware of social injustices. This worldview was a constant. Simplicity was essential to their independence: no waste, no excess, honest to word and actions. There was no place for weapons, drugs, alcohol, or cussing. There was a love for animals and all other wonders of Mother Earth. They spoke rarely, so I remember their messages to me. I loved work and as a child helped by ironing on a little board. I helped my father mix paint and saw the magic of color transform. We grew much of our food; each seed precious.

Kay Miller
*Soul Rider*
2004
78″x66″x3″
Oil on canvas and mixed media (rhinestones, wood, plastic, cotton)
Courtesy of the artist
Photography by John Bonath

Ours was an unusual household in this chemical industrial ghetto. We were the only kids in this small and impoverished neighborhood to finish high school. My parents did not have that opportunity. We were their dream realized.

I was born an activist and rebelled as I crossed borders of economic differences throughout school. The first crossing was kindergarten. Corporal punishment ruled. A lifelong poor sleeper and a sensitivity to light and sound made me lose attention easily. This was a perceived transgression, resulting in daily whippings along with kids who only spoke Spanish, which was forbidden. We were taught that we were disobedient and bad, this created unspeakable anger and fear of authority. When hearing words like "poor" and "wrong side of the tracks," I brought those questions home. Why did I have flour sack dresses? Why didn't we have a refrigerator or television? Discontent and lacking a mature social perspective, I blamed my parents. My mother knew I needed a deeper understanding and shared with me what she knew of her ancestry. The story had two parts.

I learned of a distant Comanche relative from her mother's side, Cynthia Ann Parker. She died of a broken heart. Her spirit lives in me and guides my purpose. Then I learned of the French side of my family who came here in resistance to the industrial revolution as part of a utopian colony. They called themselves the Icarians. None of these ancestors clung to either rigid identity or species-based hierarchies inherent in colonial values. Both parents were also exposed to Quaker values, influencing their commitment to non-violence. I began to connect and felt a continuum with these ancestors. Around this time, age 9, I started painting animals and flowers on clam-like shells that made up driveways.

In my mid-teens my frustration exploded in an argument with my mother that caused problems in the family. At 16, I left home forever. Deeply troubled and proud, I took full responsibility for myself, refusing help or advice. I worked a variety of low-paying jobs, saved a little money, and finished high school in summer, 1964. After I graduated, I lived in an old car, washing up at gas stations while working various odd jobs to save money for night classes at the University of Houston. These included work for a cardiologist who raped me. I never went back, but never reported it, either. Stressed and not healthy, I spent $0.25 a day for food to meet my savings goals.

In fall 1964, I enrolled at the university but soon learned that I needed an address. A dean found me one: free room and board in exchange for childcare. This offer was from an Episcopal priest and his wife, Hunter and Janet Morris. Their church was a frontline support for the Civil Rights Act and they were devoted activists. At that time, Texas was among the last states to enact the federal rulings. There was violence and turmoil in the streets.

After six years, in summer 1970, I received a bachelor of science degree, which was the same year that public schools were forced to integrate. Teachers would integrate in 1971; students in 1972. I was hired to teach in fall 1970 at an all-Black school, Jack Yates High; one with a violent history. I met great students and faculty, but as the only non-Black person, I became a target of administrators opposed to change. When faculty integrated in fall 1971, violence ensued. Things did not improve the following year when three non-Black students arrived to "integrate" a school of 1,000. This was not going well. More than 50 years later, it still isn't.

In 1970, I took part in two major events which radically defined my view of the arts. Dominique de Menil allowed me to watch her curate and place for hanging a comprehensive Magritte show from her collection at the Rice University Museum (now Moody Center for the Arts) in Houston. There I met Pauline Kael, film critic at the *New York Times,* who was teaching a semester-long class at the newly formed film studies department at Rice. These were tremendous experiences. Their visions were organic expressions of my yet still undeveloped artistic freedom. The synchronicity didn't end there.

At the same time, on a very personal level, my life was forever changed when I met Pedro. He pierced my entire reality being the most affirming person I have ever known. He showed me the pathways of open borders between art and science, beginning with the magic and mystic signs found in nature and conjured through the whole of being. My entire purpose was deeply strengthened and given direction by these timely meetings that I have carried throughout my lifetime.

Pedro expressed love in all actions. A Brahmin, a theoretical mathematician, and very primitive. Clear as a bell with the heart of a drum! His love was interior and natural. We moved to Cambridge where he took a job at MIT in 1972. Although offered, I refused a studio space. I was still troubled. I left within a year. Back in Texas, I applied and enrolled in the BFA and MFA programs at the University of Texas, Austin. This came with a studio and three years of instructor employment. During my university art education not a single woman served in painting as a professor, and there was only one non-white graduate classmate, but he left. As I looked at my future, the odds seemed stacked against me. After five years of study I received my BFA and MFA degrees in December 1978.

Seeking employment, I followed the "gypsy scholar road." Doing what I needed to survive, I accepted the lowest pay, but always insisted on having a studio. I was an inspired teacher, but what was deemed acceptable pedagogy was uninspiring. Daily, I experienced the hidden structure of systemic discrimination. I was learning that studio art departments were locked into knowledge systems tied into tenets of colonization. This is largely true today.

In 1981, I accepted a tenure-track position at the University of Iowa. This job was rewarding for many reasons, among them: the autonomous art museum. Robert Hobbs, the museum director, introduced me to an expanded world of art and I began to show my work. Participating in a show at the New Museum in New York in 1984 was rapidly followed by invitations to exhibit with Jeffrey Hoffeld, Mary Boone, and Bernice Steinbaum. Taken by surprise, I said "maybe—if I can get off work," or "I don't feel ready." I had no idea of the magnitude of these offerings. I'd painted to heal myself and hadn't considered commerce. Recognizing neither names nor timelines, I hoped to knock on their doors when ready. I remain grateful for their recognition of my work; most significantly, Jeffrey Hoffeld's observation that I was "in it for the long haul." These words carried me through many trying times to come.

At the same time, back in Iowa, an early tenure vote was held. I supported an open, inclusive view of the visual arts. Some were in full agreement, others were not. Tenure was denied based, in part, on the view by those who said I lacked an appreciation and understanding of the Western canon. As if I had not been educated by the same system as they? In 1986, I joined the University of Colorado, Boulder, where I worked for 21 years. Looking back, it is hard to fathom the years that passed. I quickly learned that I had landed in an environment lacking professionalism, and rife with both health and safety concerns for everyone. Being both new to and grateful for employment, I was slow to address these problems; but, over time, I did.

Fortunately, outside agencies and foundations continued to support my creative efforts. The Joan Mitchell Foundation, Creative Capital, P.S. 1, and others gave me experiences and personal connections forged with other creative minds that allowed my work to continue. While this support was invaluable, it was not enough to overcome events at CU that followed.

My salary was reduced—through interdepartmental machinations—to the lowest allowed for my rank. I felt unsafe and became terrified. This job culminated in a series of threats that rendered me unable to walk or speak. The involved faculty offered no assistance, mocking me as they left the room. I never painted again.

After working for decades within the university system and absent help from the administration, I sought justice through a federal lawsuit. It was filed, assigned, and ultimately abandoned when I exhausted my financial capacity. Ironically, at this same time, I earned full professor status at the university! Even that was delayed by faculty operating under the shadow of "further review." After years of cruel and intense retaliation, a mere sliver of my spirit was alive when I left in 2008 to take care of myself.

My life was heavily influenced, but not defined, by my university experiences. Fifteen years have passed since I left academia and recovery has been slow. Reflecting on my early life—so rich in the encouragement of positive life-giving and sustaining activities—further fostered by so many who showed me, through their actions, the power of love and respect in the face of injustice and indignity, I now understand that I fought the good fight. A mark was made.

Experience cannot be denied, only acknowledged and accepted. Attempts to capture anything alive are in vain. What I have tried to describe here is a part of my story; of the things I did in my attempt to continue painting. Often lacking in material means but driven by an understanding of the importance of life-sustaining activities, I created a life as a painter. In some ways, my academic career was a means to an end, driven by a need to survive. I gave of myself and expected, in return, some degree of safety and protection. I was naive.

Today, I am grateful for everything that transpired. It is all mine. I love that now I feel free to soar within a new visual form that is self-sustaining and always available; with an infinite capacity for expression. This came to me unexpectedly through my work as an artist. It was automatic, not learned or acquired, but rather induced by surprise that silenced my brain. This allowed me to return to an inner path that is inherently connected to everything that draws on the magic of life for the good of all to share.

This new self-discovery within my mind is primal in both projections and predictions of my life. It is providing clearings to make a path to enter and exit change from all directions. This started as an ontological query that led into a supernatural experience. My mind disconnected from my body and reunited with it in a rebirth of health, re-awakened spirit, and new growth from the near-death experience when I quit painting. What was intangible and invisible from my senses had bypassed my consciousness, suspending beliefs and time. This is magic. This is the purpose being revealed. Allies and angels surround me these days guiding me to free art, to free love, and to free money. ●

# MAREN HASSINGER

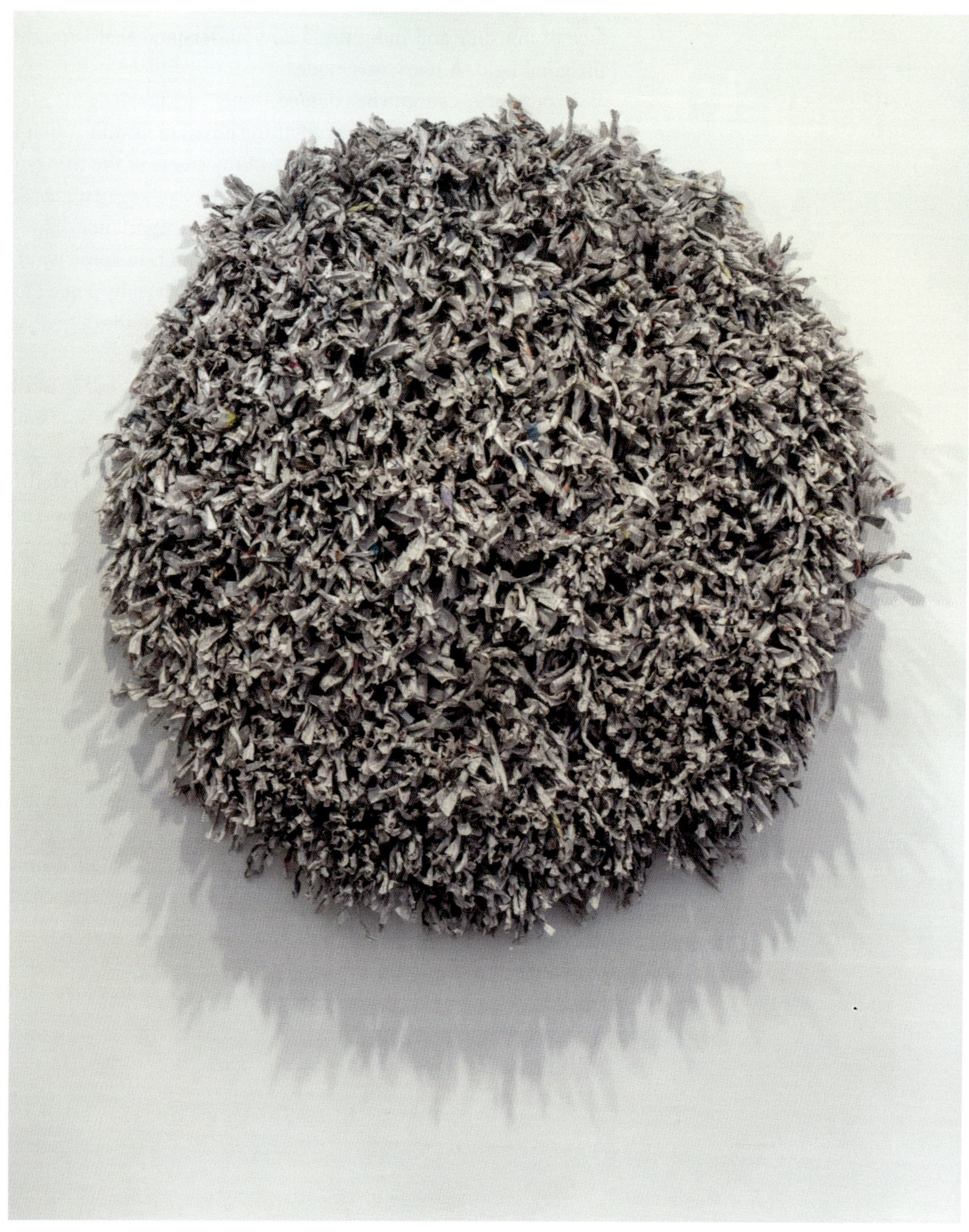

Maren Hassinger
*Our Lives*
2008–18
72″ diameter
Shredded, twisted and wrapped *New York Times* newspapers
Courtesy of Susan Inglett Gallery, NYC
Photography by Adam Reich

ARTISTIC PLATFORMS—whether autobiography, sculpture, installation, performance, fibers, film, video, photography, audience participation, light, public work, the color pink to inspire love—are all in the service of equality, our citizenship, our earth.

I didn't start out to be a visual artist. I began by wanting to dance. This was a practice I began at age 5—leaping over phone books in the creative dance classes taught by pioneers Anne and Paul Barlin. I danced more or less throughout high school, taking technique classes from Lelia Goldoni and Yvonne de Lavallade. Lelia was in the Lester Horton Dance Company with Alvin Ailey and Carmen de Lavallade. Her sister Yvonne was my teacher and in Lester's Junior Company. I also studied with Kay Turney at L.A. High. She kept us busy with innumerable performances.

In applying to Bennington College, my intention was to major in dance. My first counselor was painter Paul Feeley. He told me to take dance, art, literature, and biology. And I did! Everything was okay that first year, but when I wanted to declare as a dance major, I was denied—being told I was better in art. Anger, wrenching sadness, is what I felt. I was prepared to leave until my then counselor and drawing teacher, Pat Adams, talked me out of it. So, I stayed and majored in sculpture with Isaac Witkin (from South Africa and England), who liked a clay head I'd made.

After graduation I returned to Los Angeles and took lots of dance classes from lots of folks, including Lelia, Yvonne, and the legendary Carmelita Maracci for ballet. I also started grad school. Another disappointment, this time from UCLA's Graduate Sculpture Department. No, they said, but I was asked by Bernard Kester, who was forming a new graduate major in fiber structure, to join his group. Three years later, I became his first MFA. That was 1973. I made many things and found wire rope in a junkyard.

During grad school, I married Peter Hassinger. He is a writer I met while at Bennington when he was a student at nearby Williams College. He found a great live-in studio space on San Vicente Boulevard owned by Jay Whitehead, a painter I met at L.A. High when we were both students of Ms. Schaum. It was in this San Vicente studio that I decided to become an artist.

We wanted to have a family—children. Peter came from a devout Irish Catholic family of three children. I was an only child surrounded by suffering adults: my mother, father, and paternal grandmother. I wanted to be an artist and a mother. I did not feel they were mutually exclusive!

The phone rang one day in that studio. It was Senga Nengudi. That was the beginning of our continuing movement collaboration. We both discovered that our high school dance teachers were in Lester Horton's company. Her teacher was Jimmy Truitte, who later joined the Alvin Ailey Company.

So, L.A. was my birthplace—actual and otherwise. It all began there for me. In Camp Fire Girls—based on Native American ideology—I danced and learned about equality because there were many girls from many ethnicities. We shared each other's cultures at meetings. My grandmother was our leader and my mother was on the local committee. I learned what moving through space was. I played in a sandbox for hours on my own, sailing ships that my dad, the architect, made at University of Southern California. I learned how to negotiate authority as an only child in a family with three overachieving adults.

My life's confrontations—childhood beatings and adult disowning—are about the legacy of blackness—no laughing matter . . . It's also called genetic trauma. It's like going from nothing to nothing. We come into the world with nothing and leave with nothing. And the in-between, if you can, are choices. I was privileged in that I could make choices, even though they weren't always supported.

It was difficult to be an only child in a family of four. My dad spanked me once with his hands for staying out after school without permission, my mother (an ex-cop) spanked me with her wide, thick, black plastic policewoman's belt. She spanked me so much I couldn't remember why or how often. But I do remember the welts. She always said it was so I wouldn't get "spoiled." My grandmother Martha (who had an incredible story of abandoning her husband) was my babysitter. She "told on me." Any infraction . . . And my mother then beat me . . . All of this I blame on violent institutions like slavery and servitude. I tried my best to let this legacy stop with me. Generally, it's been easy to be a mother with kids like mine. Ava and I collaborate on art projects. My son Jesse writes beautifully and I hope someday that all of us can collaborate as well—on a film! I knew about disappointment from Bennington and UCLA. And I learned I could navigate, survive, and even excel within disappointment. I worked as an artist and teacher for 45 years before being asked to join Susan Inglett's NYC gallery. I was married for twenty years and now have two grown children, Ava and Jesse. Ava is an artist in Philly and we collaborate from time to time. Jesse works in the tech industry in San Francisco. His company makes apps to assist in Democratic political campaigns.

Life has taught me how and why to make things. It has given me a voice and a reason for being an artist. All that I feel about being black, being a woman, being a mentor, being a citizen have come to me via life. Life says make this thing to communicate. And what's most important in the world is what you believe is most needed.

So I have made many things from many materials alone and with others. And once I made the decision to be an artist, I stayed the course. That's because I believed that I had something to say. It turns out that the subject was the "loss" of nature. "Loss" is not accurate—our changing relationship to nature is a better description. Resources have dwindled and the rich and powerful have become oligarchs or created oligarchies and initiated civil wars resulting in waves of beleaguered refugees and global unrest. All land and sea resources are limited and in jeopardy. The owners' status is changing and the fight is on . . .

Making art is my way of speaking on behalf of people who cannot. My belief in the need for equality, compassion between people, and love as techniques for getting on with our lives—creating families, ending wars, working side by side—are ideas that have come to me from making art. We are citizens of the same world. In collaborative performances when audiences become performers is exactly what making is about for me. This object, this installation, these performances include all. These endless twists [see page 122] in wire rope and the *New York Times* newspapers are inspired by the umbilical cord I saw when Ava was born. Even though I had made prior twists, at her birth I SAW confirmed that this twist is common to all and binds we mammals to a similar humanity. Making things expresses all this—our unity—and the possibility for love and a life together. At the end of powwows it is said, "We are all related." •

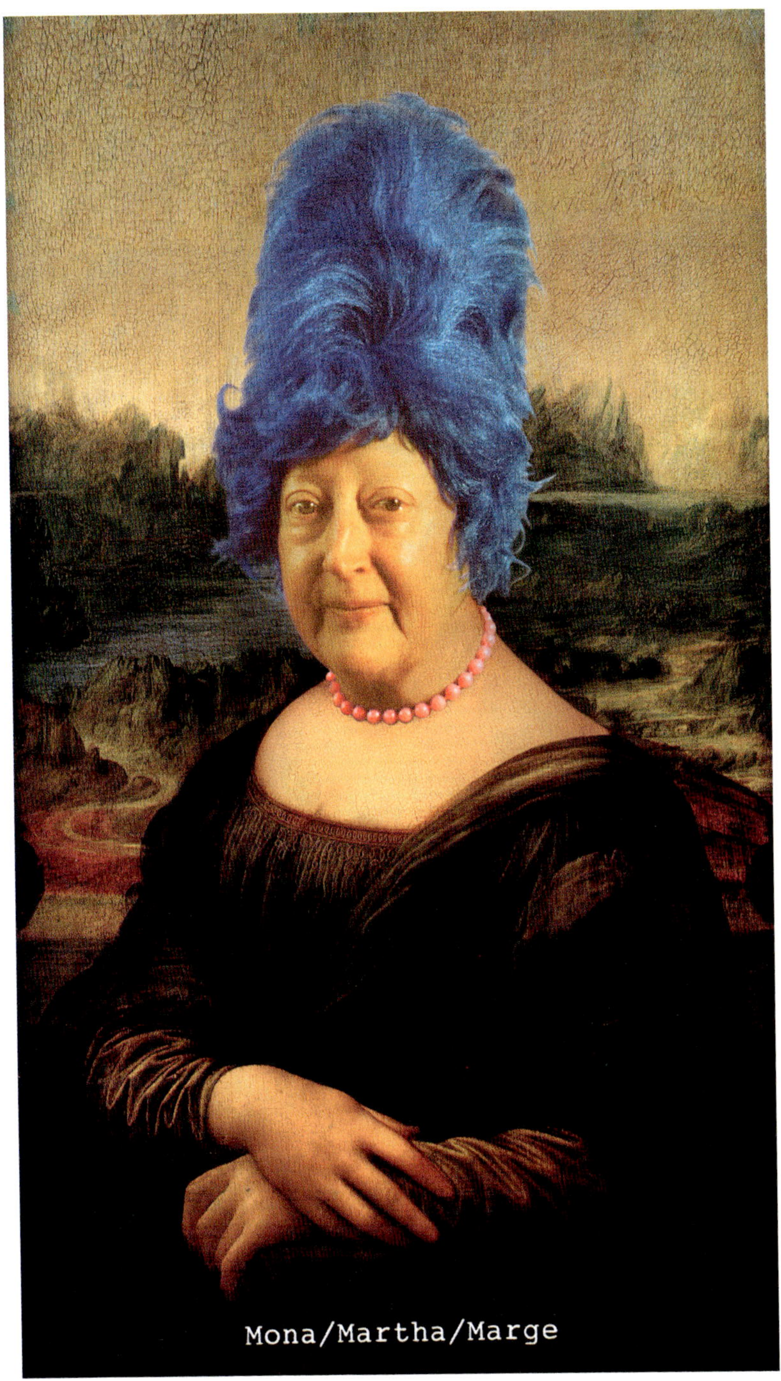
Mona/Martha/Marge

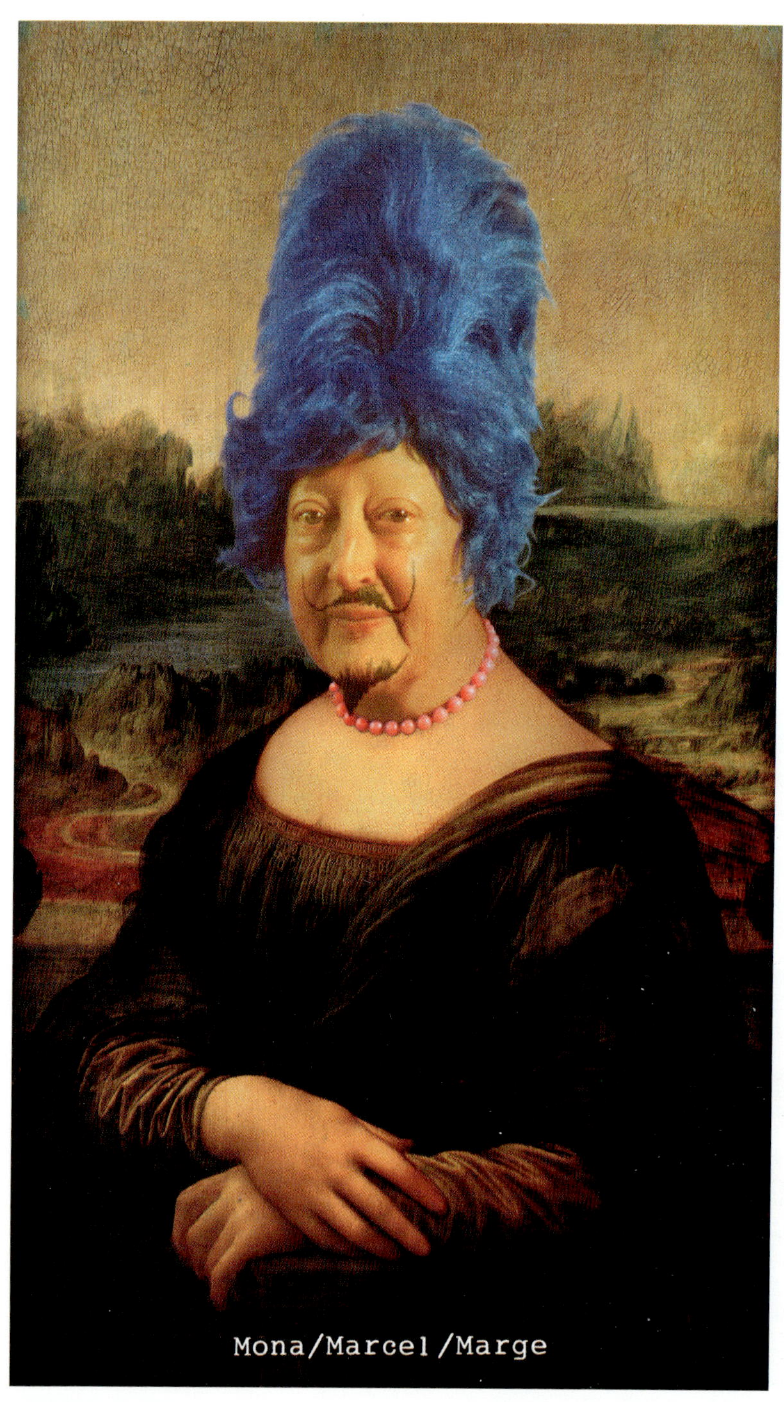
Mona/Marcel/Marge

HERE IS WHAT I wrote in my diary in 1974 after my beautiful artist boyfriend dumped my ass:

*I am drafting my own blueprint. I am writing my way out of this well. I am writing to discover an Answer. I am creating my resources out of an absence that I feel in the "real" me. All my values have been contributed from the outside, from my parents, my lovers. How do I know what "I" like, what I don't like? I let my room get messy to discover whether "I" like it that way. I listen to music to discern what "I" like. I am alone. In a panic I run to eat something sweet. I have to stop myself by force. I sit myself back down in my kitchen chair. I stare straight ahead, my right arm resting on the table. The backs of my lenses are silver; I am staring inward. I see nothing in front of me. I sip nervously at a diet soda and consciously lower my shoulders. I find muscles knotted every few minutes and have to unravel them by will. I write the same questions over and over in my diary: What do I really want to do? I am 26 and unencumbered. I have been groomed in English Literature and Art. I want to be passionately involved in something, to be able to immerse myself in something. But you don't know what you like until you do it. I am not yet able to feel my way up the wall. I will have to rationalize my way out. I will create myself into the absent center through action. Out of the building blocks floating there I will select and discard, select and*

Martha Wilson
*Mona/Martha/Marge, Mona/Marcel/Marge*
2015
29″x21″ each
Lenticular photograph
Courtesy of the artist and
P·P·O·W Gallery, New York
Compositing Artist Kathy Grove

*discard, until I have constructed an igloo, a personality. Writing will be my first brick.*

In May 1974 I moved to New York City to find out if I really was an artist. Luckily for me, I met Lynne Tillman at a party at Power Boothe's loft. She was in therapy and I wanted to be in therapy too, but I couldn't see the same therapist; so her therapist recommended Alice Entin, who, like my family, had some connections to Quakerism. I saw Alice for ten years, from 1978 to 1988, during which time I uncovered—and then blocked out—the knowledge that my father had touched me sexually when I was perhaps 6 or 7. Somewhere in the 1980s, my sister, who slept in the same room, helped me reconstruct this event. Now I believe he did this because he wanted me to be sex-positive, unlike my Quaker mother who was a "prude" in his view. But the effect of my father crossing the line from protector to predator was so traumatic that I became a bulimic; and I further believe I am an artist (and not a psychokiller) today because I had art as an outlet, a place to externalize my inner being for outside examination. What's wrong with the idea that art is therapy?

A year or so after leaving therapy I became pregnant by Scott Cook, a bartender who lived in Pennsylvania; I had met him while taking care of my mother and my mother's house in Newtown, PA. I was 40 at the time; the veil parted and I recognized that this would be my last shot at having a baby. I called Scott on the phone to tell him I was keeping the baby. He said, "You're ruining my life; I will never support you." I said, "Fine, go to hell." But at the same time, I was having horrible fears that if I had been abused as a child that I would have to abuse my own child, so I called Alice Entin for an appointment. She thankfully told me, "You can drop this torch on the ground and let it go out."

In 2017 I had my journals written from 1965 to 1983 scanned so I could find the points at which I decided to become an artist, and to found an arts organization. I read every single page, but never found the "ah-ha" moments I was looking for. The subtext of this story is that I had majored in English literature as an undergraduate, then got an MA as a graduate student at Dalhousie University in Halifax, Nova Scotia, across the street from my beautiful artist boyfriend's school, the Nova Scotia College of Art and Design (NSCAD), where he was getting an MFA in printmaking (and this being the Vietnam War era, avoiding being drafted into the U.S. Army). I would attend classes at Dal, but hang out at NSCAD because the kids were way cooler—plus, visual art was being made out of LANGUAGE by the conceptual artists invited to visit the school.

When Vito Acconci came as a visiting artist, his sexually explicit works such as *Seedbed* opened the door to sexuality as a legitimate subject of contemporary art; and the body itself as an art medium. He looked at my work and suggested I read sociologist Erving Goffman's *The Presentation of Self in Everyday Life*. In this small treatise, Goffman proposes that we are all performing all the time, for various audiences, starting with our own sense of self, then for others, then perhaps for a sense of history . . . the layers of personality were peeled away by this work, allowing me to perform my own senses of self in 1972 with videos of solo performances for the audience of the camera: "Premiere," "Routine Performance," "Art Sucks," and "Appearance as Value."

In 1971 I started making art out of language, starting with *A Short Story About Nova Scotia*, followed by *Chauvinist Pieces*. When I told my mentor at NSCAD (who had been my painting teacher at Wilmington College and had been hired away by the President of NSCAD, Garry Neil Kennedy) that I wanted to be an artist, he replied, "Women don't make it in the artworld! But if you're serious, you'll make black-and-white art." I walked across the street to the drug store and bought a roll of color film, producing *Posturing: Drag*, *Painted Lady*, and *Age Transformation* during the next couple of years.

Lucy R. Lippard, art critic, curator, and feminist activist, visited NSCAD in 1973. I showed her my work, and she said, "Yes, you are an artist. And there are other women around North America and Europe who are doing feminist work." She gave me the term "feminist" and put me in one of her "number shows," *c. 7,500*, the catalog through which I met New Yorkers Jacki Apple, Rita Myers, Alice Aycock, and Nancy Kitchel.

Because we discovered that we were interested in the same issues surrounding identity, Jacki Apple and I collaborated on a performance art work together in December 1973. It was entitled *Transformance: Claudia* and took place at the Plaza Hotel and in Soho. After I moved to New York, Jacki made an appointment for us to show our work to Ivan Karp, director of OK Harris Gallery. We showed him our stuff, and then he exploded: "Why are you showing me this work? Your work is TERRIBLE! I would never show this work!" After this trauma, I resolved to start my own arts organization, and to show 50/50 men and women (although we never really used a quota system). Jacki was curator of Franklin Furnace from 1976 to 1980, at which point she moved to Los Angeles; and Franklin Furnace established annual peer panel review of proposals which remains in place today.

In the 1970s, the not-for-profit arts organizations in Lower Manhattan were attempting to undermine the capitalist system that was embodied in the commercial galleries and uptown museums. The uptown folks were ignoring the artists' publishing movement and showing painting and sculpture. We were collecting, exhibiting, preserving, and selling artists' books; showing temporary installation works; performance art (originally called "body art," a term I like much better); fostering street actions; and generally trying to break the frame in which art had been presented for thousands of years so that it would be seen by regular people.

I started Franklin Furnace as my "day job," in the hope that I would not have to work as a waitress or secretary to support my life as an artist. (I figured if I didn't make it in the artworld I could always be a secretary again!) But that brings me to the importance of my time at Harry N. Abrams, Inc., Artbook Publishers (Abrams). When I moved to New York, I saw an ad in *The New York Times* for an editorial assistant with a background in art history and figured it was either Praeger or Abrams. I got up early, went to Abrams, and waited to speak with Margaret L. Kaplan, managing editor of the company. She was interviewing a woman who admitted she was an artist. When I saw the look on Margaret's face, I didn't mention that I was an artist—and got the job. The reason this is relevant is that while I assumed that working for Abrams would unite my interests in art and literature, what really happened was that I learned how to run a business. A few months after my arrival, Abrams decided it would be more efficient to send Margaret to Japan to proofread than to send versions of the manuscript back-and- forth across the Pacific Ocean. I was left running the editorial department! What I learned was that it is vital to have parallel systems in place so if you can't find a document you have another path. To this day Franklin Furnace keeps a "chrono file," a chronological pile of all correspondence that is sent out of the organization.

During the last four decades, Franklin Furnace has developed a place in art history for artists' books, temporary installation art, and performance art, and it has researched the history of the contemporary artists' book through such exhibitions as *Cubist Prints/Cubist Books*, *The Avant-Garde Book: 1900-1945*, *Fluxus: A Conceptual Country*, as well as thematic shows such as *Artists' Books: Japan*, *Multiples by Latin American Artists*, *Contemporary Russian Samizdat*, and *Eastern European Artists' Books*.

Franklin Furnace set upon a course of substantial change in 1993 when its collection of artists' books published internationally after 1960, the largest in the United States, was acquired by the Museum of Modern Art in New York. On September 8, 1997, Franklin Furnace sold its loft and established a cash reserve, matching in part a challenge grant from the National Endowment for the Arts.

During its twentieth anniversary season, Franklin Furnace reinvented itself as a "virtual institution" not identified with its real estate but rather with its resources, made accessible by electronic and other means. In the wake of the "Culture Wars" of the 1980s and 1990s, the organization made this decision in order to provide the artists it was presenting with the same freedom of expression possible in the loft during the 1970s. Franklin Furnace's mission statement follows:

*Franklin Furnace's mission is to present, preserve, interpret, proselytize and advocate on behalf of avant-garde art, especially forms that may be vulnerable due to institutional neglect, their ephemeral nature, cultural bias, or politically unpopular content. Franklin Furnace is dedicated to serving artists by providing both physical and virtual venues for the presentation of time-based art, including but not limited to artists' books and periodicals, installation art, performance art, and unforeseen contemporary avant-garde artforms; and to undertake other activities related to these purposes. Franklin Furnace is committed to serving emerging artists; to assuming an aggressive pedagogical stance with regard to the value of avant-garde art to life; and to fostering artists' zeal to broadcast ideas.*[1]

Like all not-for-profit cultural institutions, we are fundamentally chartered for the purpose of education. Since 1985, Franklin Furnace has hired practicing artists to work in the New York City school system under the aegis of its Sequential Art for Kids program to develop new ways for avant-garde art to serve as the basis of curriculum development.

Franklin Furnace has had an indelible impact upon art by launching the careers of artists whose work has influenced art and cultural discourse. Franklin Furnace often premieres artists in New York who later emerge as artworld stars: Ida Applebroog, Tanya Barfield, Eric Bogosian, David Cale, Cassils, Patty Chang, Willie Cole, Sue de Beer, Nicole Eisenman, Karen Finley, Coco Fusco, Kate Gilmore, Guillermo Gómez-Peña, Dustin Grella, Ann Hamilton, Mona Hatoum, Murray Hill, Jenny Holzer, Tehching Hsieh, Barbara Kruger, Shaun Leonardo, Sherrie Levine, Liza Lou, Taylor Mac, Robbie McCauley, Naeem Mohaiemen, Shirin Neshat, Rashaad Newsome, Lorraine O'Grady, Clifford Owens, William Pope.L, Liz Magic Laser, Shaun Leonardo, Emily Roysdon, Dread Scott, James Siena, Theodora Skipitares, Michael Smith, Annie Sprinkle, Krzysztof Wodiczko, and Paul Zaloom, among hundreds of others. Franklin Furnace's website reaches an international audience of every stripe, including artists, arts professionals, scholars and the general public; its social networking presence on Facebook, Twitter, Vimeo, Instagram and its blog reaches out to young audiences.

During its thirtieth anniversary season, Franklin Furnace received support from the National Endowment for the Humanities (NEH) to digitize the event archives of its first decade, and signed a collaboration agreement with ARTstor to digitize and publish on the web documentation of events it presented and produced. In 2010, Franklin Furnace received its second major grant from the NEH to digitize the event archives of its second decade, 1986 to 1996; and to publish these records on Franklin Furnace's website with the goal of embedding the value of ephemeral art practice in art and cultural history. In 2013, Franklin Furnace signed a second collaboration agreement with Artstor to enable online publication of videos of performance art works—now viewed as critical pedagogical materials.

In 2011, in order to better provide access and preserve its physical and digital archives over the long term, Franklin Furnace began a strategic planning process that resulted in the recommendation of a "nesting" relationship with an external partner to ensure the organization's continuity and cultural relevance in the twenty-first century. The timing of this strategic planning process was fortuitous, overlapping with the implementation of various academic/campus initiatives outlined in Pratt Institute's recently completed Strategic Plan. On September 30, 2014, Franklin Furnace signed an organization-in-residence agreement with Pratt, the purpose of which is to facilitate mutual pedagogical and physical access to these Brooklyn-based organizations' resources and to foster the development of ambitious collaborative projects.

Back to Martha Wilson: My friend Marvin Taylor, founder of the Downtown Collection at NYU, said that at the end of the 1970s, "Everybody was in three bands." This was certainly true for the very first members of DISBAND, Daile Kaplan and Barbara Ess (except Martha Wilson). Daile was also in Rhys Chatham's band, the Gynecologists, and Barbara Ess was in Glenn Branca's band, Static, as well as founding her own all-girl band, Y-Pants. Other bands around in the late 1970s were the Theoretical Girls, Bush Tetras, James White and the Blacks, Tone Death, Con Iced, A-Band, Daily Life, the Idiot Orchestra, the Diplomat Samurai Band, the Love of Life Orchestra. Bands played at the Mudd Club, Tr3, AREA, CBGBs, and Tonic. But they all knew how to play instruments and I didn't, so I called up artist girlfriends who were long on concept and short on skills, and in 1978, DISBAND, the all-girl band of artists who couldn't play any instruments, was born.

In Franklin Furnace I had a loft that was big enough for wild and crazy rehearsals. Honestly, we didn't rehearse all that much—mostly we gossiped and ate dinner together. In the earliest meetings, I remember April Gornik and Ingrid Sischy sitting on the floor, taking it all in. April left but Ingrid stayed. Barbara Kruger wrote two wonderful songs, "The End" and "Fashions," before leaving around the summer of 1979. Then Diane, the dancer and outspoken activist, brought in fellow live-wire Ilona Granet, a ranter in her own right and singer for Con Iced, adding a dose of "silly" to the brew. The composition of the band stabilized for awhile with Ilona Granet; Donna Henes, known by all as the Urban Shaman; Ingrid Sischy, then-editor of *ARTFORUM*; Diane Torr, and Martha Wilson, founding director of Franklin Furnace, as its members.

When DISBAND disbanded in 1982, we were playing the members of Ronald Reagan's cabinet. I did one performance in my DISBAND persona of Alexander M. Plague, Jr., one as Ronald Reagan for Soho TV, and then did Nancy Reagan for "Artists Call Against U.S. Intervention in Central America," continuing as Nancy for the remainder of Ronald Reagan's terms of office. I did Barbara Bush during George H. W. Bush's term, then Tipper Gore instead of Hillary for Bill Clinton's terms—because Tipper was booed off the stage of the MTV Inaugural Ball for implementing parental advisory language on records and CDs, and the youth of America had not forgotten.

In 2002, some of my early photo-text works were shown in *Personal & Political* at the Guild Hall Museum, East Hampton, New York. Dealer Mitchell Algus saw them, and asked if I had any more works. I took everything out from under my bed and in 2008 he showed pretty much everything in my first solo exhibition in New York. Dealer Wendy Olsoff bought *I Make Up the Image of My Perfection/I Make Up the Image of My Deformity.* A year later I asked if she would look at the work I was doing; and she asked me to join P·P·O·W Gallery. So now both my personal and professional lives have become sustainable—and it only took 50 years! •

Endnote

1 Franklin Furnace, "About Us," franklinfurnace.org website.

# MARY ADDISON HACKETT

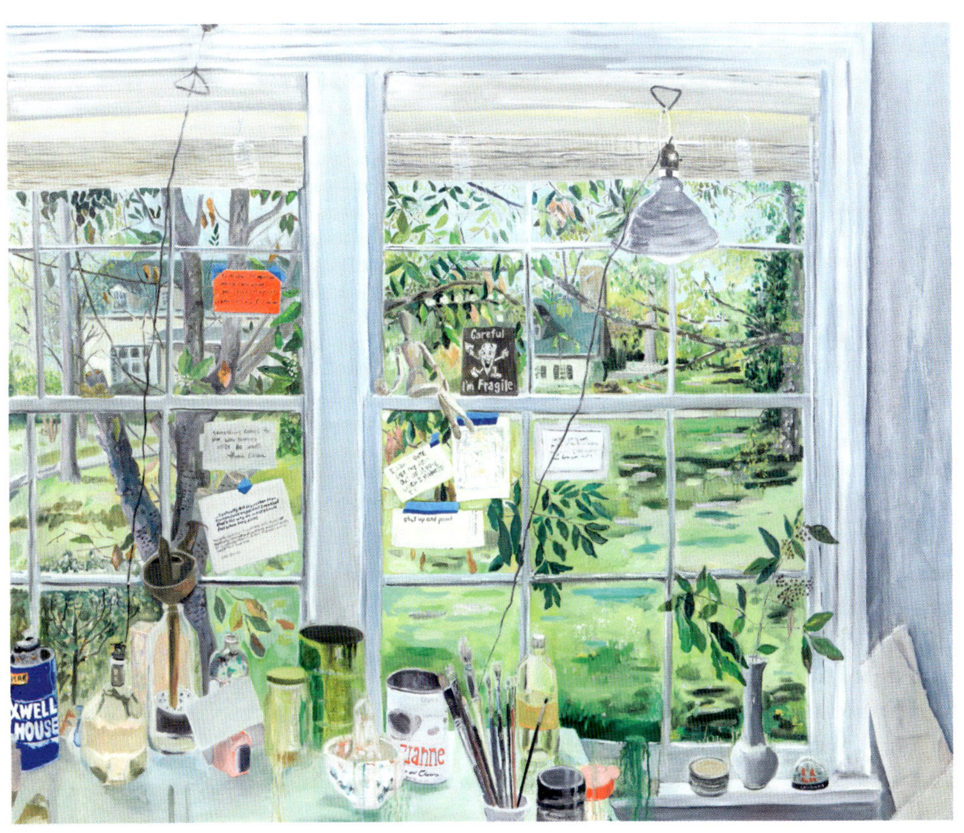

*FOLLOWING A DIVORCE, I went to see a financial consultant. When I asked if I should be worried, he replied, "Yes, and no." He then relayed that most of his clients were miserable, working at jobs they hated just so they could retire and finally live their lives—and that it looked like I, as an artist, loved what I did and seemed happy. That was the "No, I don't need to worry" part of his answer. The "yes" part was that at some point, I might have to sell my home and downsize.*

## THE SOUTH

I grew up in the 1960s and 1970s as an only child in an affluent suburb of Nashville, Tennessee. My aunt and uncle had given me a subscription to *Art in America* by the time I was 10 years old, though I had no real-life role models for how to be an exhibiting artist. I took out student loans and did my undergraduate work at the University of Tennessee in Knoxville. The visiting artist program was run by Michael Brakke, who introduced us to working artists from the East Coast. I received my BFA in painting in 1984, and after doing a residency at OxBow School of the Arts, I moved to Chicago in 1987 and set up the first of several live/work spaces.

Mary Addison Hackett
*Studio Window*
2014
54″x66″
Oil on canvas
Courtesy of the artist

## CHICAGO

Prior to attending graduate school, I supported myself through an eclectic assortment of part-time jobs and arts-related self-employment. This included everything from waiting tables and private catering, to designing gift bags for the Sara Lee Corporation, faux-finishing, sign-painting, and working as a visiting artist with adults with intellectual and developmental disabilities.

Because I anticipated the need to always have a day job, I had a work ethic of putting my arts practice first. By the time I entered grad school, it was the early 1990s and I had stopped painting. After reading *Essays on the Blurring of Art and Life* by Allan Kaprow, I began paying attention to ordinary moments and developed a post-studio practice documenting my life at home. I received a workshop grant from P.O.V. Television and my grad school advisor planted the seed that to pay the bills and have access to equipment, I could support myself as a film editor. I received my MFA in studio arts from the University of Illinois at Chicago in 1995 and eventually landed a full-time staff position as a commercial film editor at the now-defunct Chicago post house, Avenue Edit. It was a creative, high-pressure environment and I gained invaluable business skills that carried over into my life as an artist. The owner let us work on our own projects, and I was happy screening my experimental films at underground film festivals and working on documentary projects. Other than a few group shows, I had drifted away from pursuing commercial galleries.

## LOS ANGELES

In 2000, I moved to Los Angeles (L.A.) with my then-partner and soon-to-be ex-husband, a film editor I had met while living in Chicago. The following year I lost my job as an editor and with it, access to in-kind post-production services. I rented a studio in a building with other artists, started painting again, and began teaching studio art courses in the California Community College system. My network expanded organically through studio visits, residencies, and exhibition opportunities.

Because I'm introverted and socially awkward, I had to find ways to connect that worked for me. As part of my practice, I also wrote and still do today. In 2005, I began publishing a diaristic art blog called "Process." Through the blog, I struck up a correspondence, and later a friendship, with Sharon

Butler at *Two Coats of Paint*. (Fast forward, and I'm still an occasional contributor.)

At the age of 47, I had my debut solo show with the now-defunct Kristi Engle Gallery in L.A. Art Critic Christopher Knight reviewed the show in the *Los Angeles Times* and I was optimistic about having rebooted my career as a painter. On the flip side, the show opened during the 2008 financial crisis. Nothing sold, and thanks to the California state budget crisis, most of my classes were canceled. I was also managing long-distance eldercare. A divorce was imminent and I made plans to move back to Nashville to help my mom. In 2010, our home in L.A. went into escrow the day my mom passed away. Two weeks later, I moved across the country to live in my childhood home in Nashville while I sorted things out.

## NASHVILLE

When I first arrived in Nashville, I was still showing in Los Angeles, but I also wanted to be involved in the local arts community. I started teaching college-level studio art classes again as an adjunct, joined COOP, a curatorial collective, and did some arts writing. Mery Lynn McCorkle, a Georgia-based artist who I first met in L.A., curated my work into a show in Brooklyn, which led to a couple of other shows in New York and eventually a solo show with the Marcia Wood Gallery in Atlanta. When Dane Carder invited me to curate a show in his artist-run space, threesquared, I hosted several out-of-town artists whose work I wanted to bring to Nashville. Regionally, art writers supported my work, and I occasionally wrote about other artists' work for *Two Coats of Paint* and locally, *Locate Arts* and the *Nashville Scene*.

By 2015, I was nearing the end of producing a major body of work that was physically and emotionally heavy for me, and I wanted to get back to a lighter practice. I had a solo show which had been difficult to navigate. My home in Nashville was considered a teardown, which made for a great studio, but was becoming costly to maintain. I was frustrated with the universal treatment of adjunct teachers and wanted to re-up my skill set to make myself more employable. I circled back to working with lens-based media. It started with straight photography and evolved into a series of filmed conversations with women artists I knew. Although the project was a labor of love, I used it as an opportunity to update my editing skills. Looking back it sounds like a laundry list of sorrows, but at the heart of it, I was still processing the loss of my last parent and adjusting to life back in my hometown. By the time the 2016 election rolled along, the political landscape of the South was much more conservative than I had remembered and at the time I didn't see how I could effect change. I sold my childhood home in 2017 and after talking with some artist friends in L.A. who had studios in the high desert, I bought a small house in a rural area of Joshua Tree, California.

## THE MOJAVE DESERT

Initially, I moved to Joshua Tree somewhat intending to pick up my career in Los Angeles where I left off. Being roughly 90 minutes from downtown L.A. with no traffic, it was an affordable option to city living. Instead, I took on the role of a rural homesteader, fell in love with the solitude that comes with remote desert living, and rarely left.

In the desert, my income came from various sources that helped establish me in the local arts community. I pitched essays to *Two Coats of Paint* about the arts in Joshua Tree, which led to meeting artist/curator Bernard Leibov and later, an invitation from Bernard to participate in the 2019 Joshua Treenial with a site-specific video project. I picked up some documentary production work and from there, I joined the board of Arts Connection, a regional arts organization, facilitated a series of contemporary artist lectures at Joshua Tree National Park, and taught painting and photography at the local college. While in the desert, I was also fortunate to work with John O'Brien on some of his curatorial projects in L.A. Prior to leaving Nashville, I became friends with artist Vesna Pavlović, and we've since recommended one another for opportunities.

The South, Again.

I thought I would stay in the desert indefinitely, but during the 2020 pandemic solitude turned into isolation. To cope, I began documenting nearly every aspect of my life trying to make sense of what was going on in the world. My social life consisted of going to the post office and teaching on Zoom.

During the semester break, I had a profound sense of longing to return "home"—even though there was no physical space to return to. I missed the landscape of my upbringing and wanted to make work that was more directly rooted in that experience. As a result of the 2020 presidential election, I was also excited by the progressive social change happening in the South. I celebrated my 60th birthday in the desert and moved back to Nashville in late 2021.

When I moved back South this time, I did so knowing I might be operating further outside the artworld in my origin story, but closer to who I am as an artist. My solo exhibition of screen-based works opened last weekend at Unrequited Leisure in Nashville and I was bowled over by the support of friends and strangers. Since moving back I've been invited to speak about my practice as an artist to MFA students at both Vanderbilt University and Belmont University, and I was anonymously nominated for the Joan Mitchell Fellowship grant. When I lived here before, my goals were different and I expected everything to work like it had in L.A. For numerous reasons, it doesn't, and I now see that as a plus.

I have a diaristic practice documenting mostly mundane situations in and around my home, and since the early 1990s, I've worked at folding my art and life into one another. Being receptive to change, combined with living and working in different parts of the country, has shaped my practice in ways I never planned. I keep my overhead low, and I live simply. Luck and timing in real estate alleviated some immediate financial stress, but life is fragile and circumstances can change overnight. When I reflect my work as a whole, I see a clear pattern of intention driven by curiosity. I love my life and I believe in the work. ●

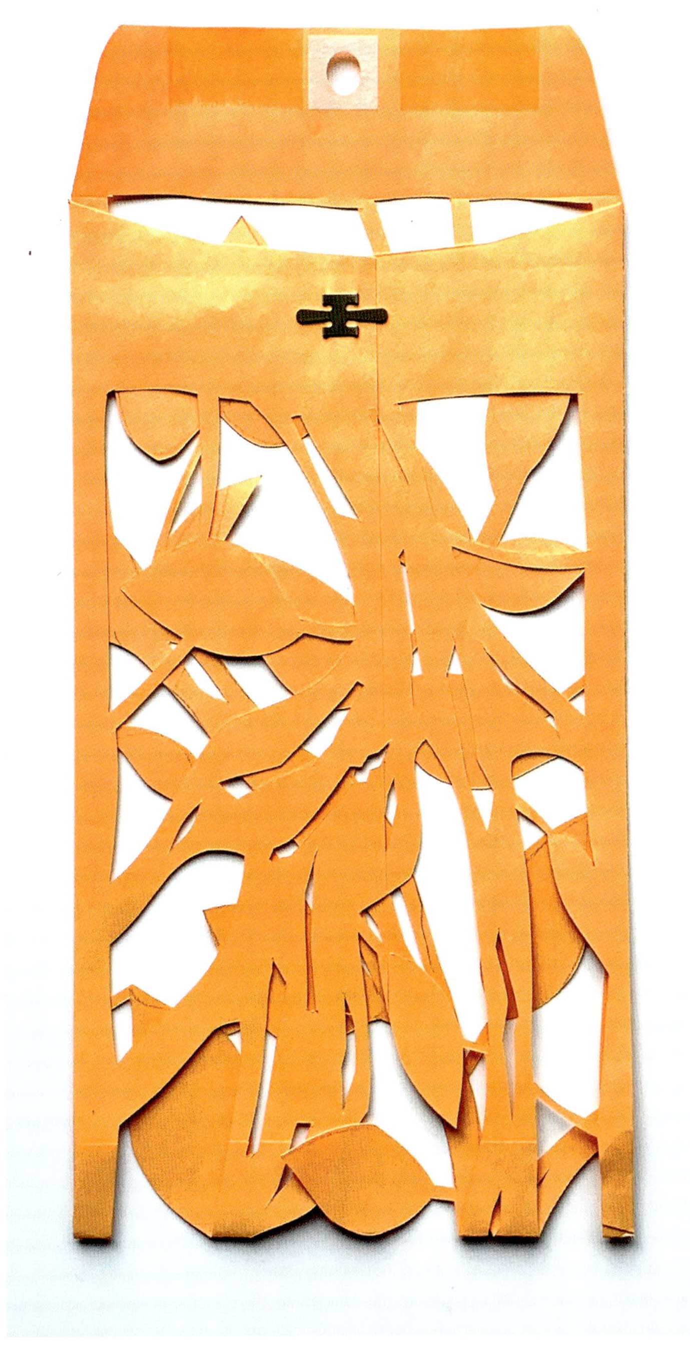

*A FILIPINA AND a German walk into a bar.*

This isn't a joke. It's the beginning of me meeting Joachim in Atlanta, Georgia, then falling in love as 23- and 26-year-olds in 1993. A mutual friend had invited us both to practice our German at the local Taco Mac over imported beer and Buffalo wings. At that age, I had a BA in psychology from University of California Berkeley and was still trying to find my way. As an immigrant born in the Philippines who grew up in Germany, Israel, and the United States, I wasn't used to planning my life long term, but rather living in the moment and making the best out of it.

Joachim was freshly diagnosed with a rare muscular disease and got through law school. We both connected deeply with each other because I had lost my father and Joachim, his sister, to suicide. Intrinsically optimistic and bright eyed, we didn't know where our lives would take us, but we knew we would care for one another.

In 1994, after selling most of my belongings, including my guitar, for a one-way ticket to Germany to be with him, I didn't know I was about to enter the artist's life. Between 1994–2000, through twists and turns (brief stint in medical school, marriage, miscarriage, then baby), Joachim saw me burning out. We were living in a small apartment in Munich, Germany, and he encouraged me to sign up for a weekend art workshop

Mic Dino Boekelmann
*Narra I*
2022
14″x10″
Manila envelope
Courtesy of the artist

at the local adult school. After picking up my first paintbrush, something ignited in me and I started churning out paintings.

I used canvas to cover up my toddler room's floor as a makeshift home studio. At night I played Ennio Morricone's *The Mission* soundtrack to get me into the right mood. Meanwhile, Joachim found a rental space for me to exhibit my work in Munich at the Sardenhaus, which was situated in a public park. Deadlines make me super-efficient and I made sixteen large paintings in three months to fill the three rooms, designed the invites, and biked around to hang up posters for the show. From carving out my own studio in our two-bedroom apartment to having conversations with the public about their thoughts around my art, it was deeply satisfying; selling ten paintings was a bonus too.

The drive and direction for art emerged in a big way, but I knew I needed more language and tools to be able to convey the ideas that were inside of me. I ventured to make my own art curriculum which would work for me and my little family, which I prioritized. I was 30 years old, a late starter now committed to what I imagined could be an artist's life.

After living in Munich, we moved to a townhouse in the suburbs of New Jersey in 2001, right after 9/11, due to Joachim's job and then I had my second miracle kid after going through another miscarriage and fertility treatments. These experiences have taught me quickly to remain flexible with plans, goals, and timeframes. I had to figure out what "regular" or "consistent" meant for my lifestyle. Once I let go of the conventional terms and descriptors, my practice had the freedom to define itself.

Although juggling the many responsibilities as a caregiver for my family, like picking up my 6-year-old son from school while nursing a newborn, it still gave me some flexibility to pursue my cobbled-together art education. Joachim's muscle disease, myotonic dystrophy, started showing up officially with weakness in his hand. Since there is no cure for it yet, it would progressively affect other parts of his body. We needed to stay flexible as every day came with new challenges. Taking art workshops taught by local artists in the area and committing to three years of atelier training in painting, it took me around ten years to get the tools I felt I needed to pursue my artistic endeavors. This fit my schedule and I learned to trust my pace. Everything became studio spaces in the house: basement, dining room table, and bedrooms. My kids were used to seeing my art all over the place. They lived with it daily and knew it had a respectful place in our home. I never forced them to partake in it, unless they were curious and wanted to know something about a certain technique. In hindsight, I do think it influenced how they viewed life: creativity is not a separate entity but an inherent part of being human.

In 2011, after a couple of women in my circle asked me to teach them how to draw and paint, I came up with an art class—The Art Getaway—that I would've enjoyed as a late starter, and it included cappuccinos during breaks. In 2013, I was hired to teach art to kids from pre-K to eighth grade at Princeton Day School, a private school nearby, as I continued giving art classes at home and still being the primary caregiver of my family.

Professionally, I set various goals for myself, for example producing 40 paintings by the age of 40 after having a dream where I died and wandered in the room where people were grieving. All I could think of as I looked at the walls was: "That's it? That's all I made? That's not enough art." In order to accomplish this by the time I got to work at my 8:00 a.m. teaching job at the school, I would wake up at 4:00 a.m. and sit at my dining table and paint. On the weekends, I rented a shared art space with four other women I had met through art classes in order to stay in touch with other artists.

I thought I was on my way toward completing my goals by cramming into my schedule as much art as possible to compensate for my late entry into the professional artist's journey. No one gave me a template on how to go about it, so I inevitably tried the usual things it takes to be an artist, like taking part in exhibitions and connecting with other artists in the area. But when I thought I had finally developed a structure for myself, my family, and my practice, by trying to do all of it and at the same time, it pretty much dissolved in 2015 when I had to go through brain surgery for hemi-facial spasm and was put on three weeks of bed rest afterwards. I believe this was caused by burnout.

*While my surgeon's hands were probably not insured like Marlene Dietrich's legs, for me they were worth $$$$$. Not only did he go into the deepest part of my brainstem and fix the spasm I had developed, but the surgery also gave me the biggest revelation for my art career.*

In 2020, since turning 50, it finally dawned on me that the beauty of getting older is accumulating an enormous amount of data to evaluate my life. My body had given me a big fat warning sign saying: "If you want to continue, you need to slow down and respect me."

I needed to change the structure of my art practice and my life in general. Until then, I've always had migraines and cramps that were worse than childbirth labor. I thought it was normal to lose days and live with pain. So it probably didn't register when my body said "enough." I was stuffing my schedule with all sorts of responsibilities because I thought I needed them to get ahead. Now I join artists with unconventional paths who are willing or forced to tweak their lifestyle so they can continue creating art long term.

Presently, Joachim's muscle disease has been manifesting in significant ways, so much so that at one point he will need a wheelchair to get by, so I need to further adjust my life as an artist and as his care partner at the same time. Now that I'm 52, I'm very protective of my energy. I love collaborators who are thoughtful—that means clear communication, mindful planning, and uplifting energy. I'm really too old for games and general dumbfuckery, which as I know now, were already a complete waste of time in my 20s, 30s, and 40s.

For some, slowing down is agony. For me, it's nurturing my health and my loved ones for the long game. It meant taking a break from painting and using manila envelopes as my medium when I found out I had a significant percentage of cadmium in my blood. It means being smart, taking inventory of what's working and not working, then proceeding forward with care.

*"Don't stress it, press it," describes the gadget Joachim bought me.*

It's called an Easy Button and when you press it, it blurts: "That was easy!" in a mechanical tone. When it comes to applying for opportunities or emailing people who don't know me, I still feel anxious that I will be rejected or what not. This is where the Easy Button comes in. I press it once I finish a task that I thought was hard. It creates an air of lightness for me, prevents me from overthinking, and gives me a token pat on the back.

Since 2018, I've gotten excited by finally seeing applications succeed like being accepted to the Creative Capital Professional Development Program, the New York Foundation for the Arts (NYFA) Immigrant Artist Program and the Chautauqua School of Art Residency. All of these have been instrumental in changing my artistic direction for the better. And with each opportunity, my confidence grows. If you would've told me twenty years ago that I was going to be instrumental in nurturing relationships within the Filipino-American art community on the east coast and hosting weekend artist residencies at my own studio, I would not have believed you. But here I am.

As an extroverted hermit, I actually love my couch, but I value being grounded in community as well. Consequently, a super important thing was connecting with other like-minded Filipino artists. The Easy Button and the Filipino American Artist Directory (founded by Janna Añonuevo! Salamat!) came in handy. I wrote to many artists living in New York, New Jersey, and Pennsylvania and invited them to my home. Surprisingly, I received a positive response and a group of us met, sat around my dining table, ate Filipino food, and discussed our backgrounds and challenges we had as artists. This was the start of my intentional efforts to create deep relationships within my community.

Out of these talks emerged the Filipino American collective NExSE, Northeast by Southeast. And this all happened right before the 2020 pandemic lockdown. We met regularly and experimented with virtual collaboration like videoing ourselves playing Filipino hackysack (*sipa*) and splicing them together.

Since then we have managed to cultivate conversation around our different Filipino-American experiences through public programming and shows at Princeton University and the NARS Foundation on Governors Island in New York.

*I ensure I'm on vacation everyday—even if it's only for fifteen minutes.*

It's having morning coffee with Joachim that makes me happy. We discuss work, fears, plans, fun, and dreams. We usually make each other laugh. This is grounding and joins a myriad of activities I do to ready myself for the day like breathing techniques or weeding the yard. There are just too many inevitable shitshows that have and will happen, so preparation to center myself and get my daily dose of joy is key for me. Art is a long game that I want to be part of and it has been proven that Joyful Mic can sustain the game more than Burned Out Mic.

My home and attached studio have become sacred. When we could renovate our house to eliminate stairs and make it more accessible for disabled folks like Joachim, I became really interested in sharing my art space with others. I signed up for a three-day workshop in 2020 on creating residencies and one of the participants, Alessandra Santos Pye, reached out to me via email to meet regularly and take the steps to make our ideas happen.

Artists Marnie Temple and Felicia Holman soon joined and after several Zoom rooms we all decided to fly out to British Columbia to a beautiful residency Marnie and her partner Jim founded called the Empire of Dirt. This was the beginning of the BIPOC Emerging Residency Leadership Collective (ERL). Each one of us created a different iteration of an art residency with the common denominator being the culture of care. These three women activated the confidence in me to host my first micro-residency in 2022. As written about in the online publication *Hyperallergic*, its focus is on rest and recalibration, something I believe every artist needs these days, including myself.

I see myself creating art and being part of uplifting creative communities for a very long time to come. Starting a little later than others in my life has just given me more fire to stay on my own course, build healthier structures for artists, and collaborate with those not typically represented. I know now that I don't have to compromise my body nor my care for loved ones to be able to do that. My children are now 24 and 18, both have seen me through my highest and my lowest. Since they were little they have attended my exhibits and to this day, having left our home for work and university, they continue to support me and give me valuable feedback on my work with an intergenerational perspective. This family has always been proud of me and has taken my career as an artist seriously. They provide the stability that I need as I determine my next steps as a professional artist. •

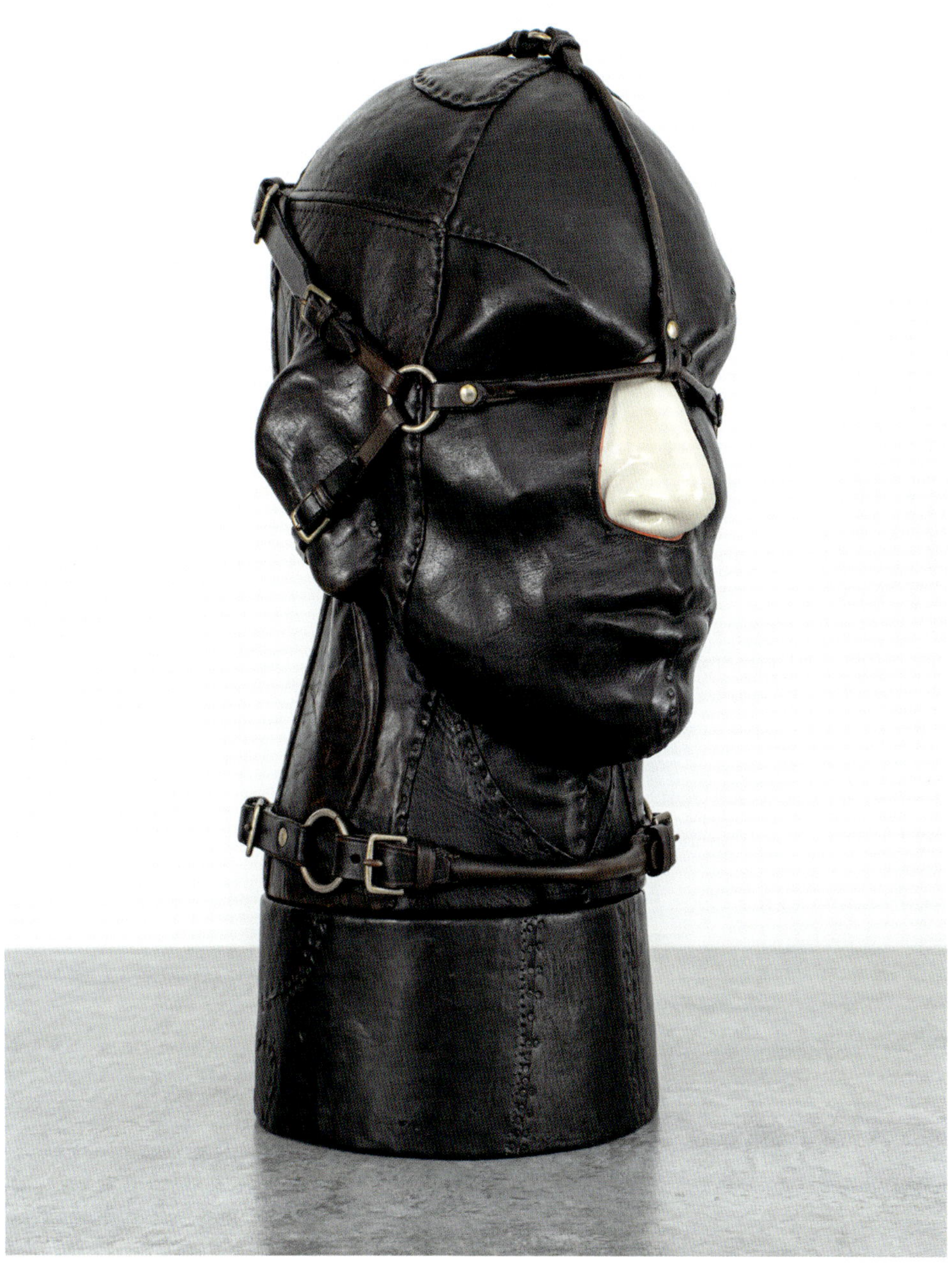

IN 1957, WHEN I was only 17 years old, I began art school at Pratt Institute in Brooklyn, New York, on an academic scholarship. I had to work my way through school, because my parents were not financially able to help me, although sometimes they did. There was a kind of admiration for my artistic abilities and some kind of support. When I was a child, my aunts, uncles, cousins, siblings, and parents used to gather around me and watch as I would draw a pocket, then a hand in the pocket, then the arm, then the jeans, then the boots, until I had a whole drawing of a cowboy. They were mesmerized, as if I were performing a magic trick. It was something I did that made me very special to the other children and my parents. I'm sure that's why I became an artist.

At that time, in the 1950s, Pratt Institute didn't even have a fine arts department. They were known for their library school and their engineering school. The closest thing I could get to being an "artist" was a department called "graphic arts and illustration." It was only when I met people who were actually studying with Abstract Expressionist painters who taught at Pratt at night (I attended Pratt as a matriculating student during the day) that I realized there was such a thing as the secret life of the painter. I mean, for me it was a secret life. I had a boyfriend who attended Pratt at night on the G.I. Bill. He used to come home and challenge me with all the problems that his teachers, Adolph

Nancy Grossman
*J*
1979–80
17″x8 3/8″x9 1/4″ /
43.2x21.2x23.5cm
Leather, wood, paint, epoxy and metal hardware
Signed
© Nancy Grossman
Courtesy of Michael Rosenfeld Gallery LLC, New York, NY
Photography by Michael Rosenfeld Gallery LLC

Gottlieb and Larry Calcagno, would give him during his classes. They were special problems. They were Abstract Expressionist vocabulary problems. And I would fail miserably. But it was an orientation to constructing and solving spatial problems in the work, which in a way I still have. Even though I use big heavy materials, very often my approach has to do with accident and discovery.

While I was at Pratt, I met a couple of people who were very influential in my life. One of them was a German-born painter teaching at Pratt named Richard Lindner. He was very smart and wonderful with students. I remember how startled I was to hear him reveal a European class bias about the lower status of those "other" artisans who worked with their hands. These were the tailors, shoemakers, carpenters, jewelers, and bakers whose hands became calloused, soiled, and sore. Lindner was a child musical prodigy who gave concerts across Europe, and he considered the three Ps—pianist, poet, and painter—superior to sewing, stitching, and struggling with the physical world of heavy burdens and endless tasks. I was bemused to think of all the adults in my extended family who worked with their hands. He was also one of the few people who wasn't particularly sexist. Maybe he was, in his personal life, but on a very deep, personal artistic level, his contention was that his best, most creative students were women. He thought it was kind of tragic that they would get married, have children, and stop painting. By the time I finished Pratt in 1962, I already knew. I was painting and painting. I was going to be an artist. It was very straightforward.

And I was very clear about what to do. You needed to pay your rent and you needed materials. And your work was going to bring you those things. So there was no problem searching for a dealer, starting at one end of Madison Avenue, which was filled with galleries in those days, in the early 1960s. I went to every single gallery with a portfolio of drawings and a couple of slides and things. I wasn't the least bit interested in "Gee, you're good," or "You're not good." It was irrelevant to me. When I think about the places I walked into and how ultimately inappropriate they were, I laugh. I wouldn't say I was an overly secure person, but I had a sense of conviction about my work. When I finally walked into what seemed like the 9,998th place, the Oscar Krasner Gallery, Oscar said, "You got any drawings?" He was very condescending. "Your drawings are really nice, kid. Your paintings? I can't show your paintings. I'll take the drawings, but not the paintings." I said, "If you take my work, you have to take all of it." I'd stubbornly maintained that position until very recently, when I realized it's a waste of my energy, and who cares anyway? It's saying, "Love me, love all of me. Love my dog, love my landscapes." But today, everything has changed so much, that if you have some red paintings and some blue paintings and someone is interested in only the red ones, I don't know, maybe it's all right to just show red paintings, then.

I think young artists today experience a burden, an overload, because being an artist has become a viable endeavor. It became recognized sometime in the mid-sixties as a "profession." Artists began to appear with models in the pages of *Vogue* and *Harper's Bazaar*. It's the cult of personality now. It's OK to be an artist. People began to imitate artists. And somewhere during that time (the mid-1960s), Americans began collecting American art in a big way. The collectors and museums and the artists began to make it a viable profession.

My deeply-held conception was that when you're an artist, you're not competing with other artists down the street. You're competing with all of art history and you're competing with yourself. Your own best efforts. That's what you have to get better than. And you have to get better than Michelangelo, you have to get better than Rembrandt. You have to get better than the very best there ever was that ever made the visual gift to all of civilization. You take everybody on. Until you love your work so much that you feel you're really making a big breakthrough with your own work, it's worthwhile to try to make money at another job entirely away from art.

In the early 1960s, I lived and set up my studio in a small storefront in the depressed part of Little Italy, in lower Manhattan. I did odd jobs in order to pay my rent and do my work. A friend offered me an illustration job which was beneath his consideration because it didn't pay well enough (12 illustrations for $150), but it was better than what I was getting paid for painting stores and apartments. Instinctually, I felt very threatened, like I would be compromised and seduced by making "a lot of money" at something that was not my real desire and my love, but still "art-ish." Nevertheless, a friend from Pratt suggested I meet a certain agent that paid better. I went to see her with my portfolio and she hired me. I illustrated many text books and short stories for her. But I never got my passion involved. I treated them at sort of arm's length.

I had my first solo exhibition at the Krasner Gallery in New York City in 1964, when I was 23 years old. The critical attention was immediately good. And even though the whole show sold out (the prices were very modest), I can't say I could support myself because, I couldn't. Brian O'Doherty from the *New York Times* gave me a wonderful review. You could say that was a success, in relation to what artists expected in those days.

In 1965, I had applied for, and won, a John Simon Guggenheim Memorial Foundation Fellowship in Painting for $5,000. When my illustration agent found out that I had won a Guggenheim she was horrified and stopped getting work for me because she only hired illustrators, not painters (because at that time artists were considered "the great unwashed"). But that was fine with me, the fellowship gave me the luxury of time to work in my studio on my own work. I didn't have to worry about paying the rent and having all these odd jobs. It was so heady and so exciting. But suddenly my acknowledged "official identity" was as a "painter" and the specificity of the designation was threatening to me. So much of growing and moving ahead in your life has to do with permission (especially if you're a woman). It felt claustrophobic. I had to make room for myself, so I immediately stopped painting. I came off the canvas and into the room. I started making huge three-dimensional construction collages with found materials. The stretcher bars I had formerly prepared for paintings, I now fronted with plywood, over which I stretched white canvas. I proceeded to make action drawings of machine/animal figures and build form using metal, plastic, wood, leather, and rubber, interchangeably "sewn" together with galvanized wire. They were huge, spontaneous action drawings/paintings; animated in space, physically overpowering, energetic, yet formally elegant. Those months in the studio were like being in love; my work was my lover. And I wouldn't leave the scene. Every day was like going out to play as a child, totally absorbed, disappeared, but completely powerful. One discovery led to another. Oh ecstasy! Sometimes I was invisible, for hours, sometimes days and nights. It was one of the most productive times in the studio; I had produced enough work for two separate exhibitions.

When the money from the Guggenheim came to an end, I reapplied for another, but they didn't grant second fellowships. So I had to go out with my portfolio (this time without the aid of an agent), to see children's book publishers directly, and find myself more illustration jobs. I took on five different children's books to do. I calculated that they would each take me just a month or two to complete. But they dragged on and on. And I was sitting at my kitchen table doing them, not in my studio, where I had left everything just where it was (one piece half finished.)

With my own work, I was always standing. This is very important because it changed my whole metabolism. I got slower and slower. The noisy exuberance and physicality of the work I had left in my studio was gone. It was more than nine months before I finished those illustration jobs, and now at least, I had bought myself time. But when I walked back into the studio, I no longer recognized the work I'd left behind. I wasn't the same person. I had become quiet and deliberate and I didn't know *who* had been doing all this noisy, energetic, dynamic work before. All I had had in my hand for nine months straight was a pencil or a rapidograph pen. But even so, I had done two years' worth of illustration work in nine months. And I had changed in the process. I started making drawings of the "state" I was in, in a figurative way. Little tiny drawings, one after another. I felt very secretive about them, because they were really self-portraits. And those were the drawings that eventually led me to the head sculptures. So I had bought myself a year in my studio. I had given myself my own Guggenheim.

The imagery in my drawings was so compelling to me that I needed to make them more profoundly real in the physical world.

But I needed to find materials that I could move around and drastically change as the work developed. The only sculptural material that answered my needs was wood. I began to make these head sculptures. They were wooden sculptures, which I carved with carpenter's tools, not sculptor's tools (I had never formally learned how to carve or sculpt). I had to think about it a lot. I decided they needed to have their own skin. And I used skins. I used leather. They weren't like voodoo dolls or anything like that. They felt completely, tremendously right to me. Each one led me to another one, the same as my paintings had before. Every painting had had some unsolved, uninvestigated problem that it opened up. And the same with these sculptures. It was a time of deep, obsessive involvement with the work. These images were very primary to me. They were really self-portraits.

In 1968, I was still officially with the Krasner Gallery when I began to do these drawings that led me to do sculpture. I went to see Oscar Krasner, having done all this work and not having shown him any of it. I said to him "I want you to sell my work so that I have enough money to pay my rent and buy materials. I don't want to do illustrations anymore. I don't want to have to stop working in my studio to do odd jobs." He said, "What do you want, kid? Egg in your beer?" I was really depressed. (Krasner's solution was always that I should teach, like so many other artists he knew did. But, I knew that because I am very much an "all in" person, I would become too invested in teaching and I wouldn't have anything left over for my own work.) He said, "Alright. If you can find somebody that can do better than me, good, go, go. You're free!" And I said, "Okay." I had these fabulous sculptures at home that I had done and not shown anybody. I decided I was going to find a different gallery. It was a big challenge. So I went to Arne Ekstrom, who was Richard Lindner's art dealer at the time and in whose gallery I had seen a variety of different artists whose work was more personal. He was very good. When he finally decided to handle my work, he made it very visible. Out of his gallery, Cordier and Ekstrom, it became very collected. He was cautious with price, so there was nothing to get rich about right then and there. But it led to tremendous visibility. You can't say that you're rich and famous these days, but you can be famous without being rich—sadly enough.

The sudden "fame" made me very self-conscious. And it completely put into jeopardy my secret life as an artist, because now it was a "public life". In some way it was open to the public, because in just one year, my work was EVERYWHERE. *Vogue Magazine, Time Magazine, Newsweek Magazine, New York Magazine, Harpers Bazaar Magazine, Art in America, Art News, Art Forum, Art's Magazine, Village Voice, New York Times.* It was very hard to integrate this new visibility. And I wasn't ready for that amount of exposure. I had to grow up. My work went ahead of me, in the sense that it ANNOUNCED who I was before I actually KNEW WHO I WAS, and I had to grow into my work. All the repercussions of the visibility challenged me and nearly crushed me in some ways. And I think that happens to everyone in that situation. I was connecting to people in a way I didn't realize at the time. Because, once again, my work was very connected to me.

Having a personal life was always dependent on the time and the needs. If the need was to have a child, then that would have been the most important thing. I would have taken the time out to do it. I work the same way. I work out of need. I'm a very unserene person. There are times in my life when my vulnerability, internal landscape, and world outside reached a kind of balance. Not a harmony, mind you, but quite the opposite. And for many years, the most exquisite feeling I could experience was when I was deeply involved in my work. I didn't exist anymore. Only what I was doing existed. You might assume that my conscious life was painful, and yes, in some ways it was. Now, having lived longer and having had to deal with these realities, I find my everyday life less painful and I find it more difficult to find uninterrupted time alone in my studio.

The important part of "still standing" is that I've had to constantly adjust to my income throughout my life. Now, at 84 years old, I am fortunate to have financial stability, good health, reliable assistance, loyal, supportive friends and family and art dealers I trust and adore. But I still live by the sweat of my brow, by my work, and I've always answered, and still answer, only to myself. •

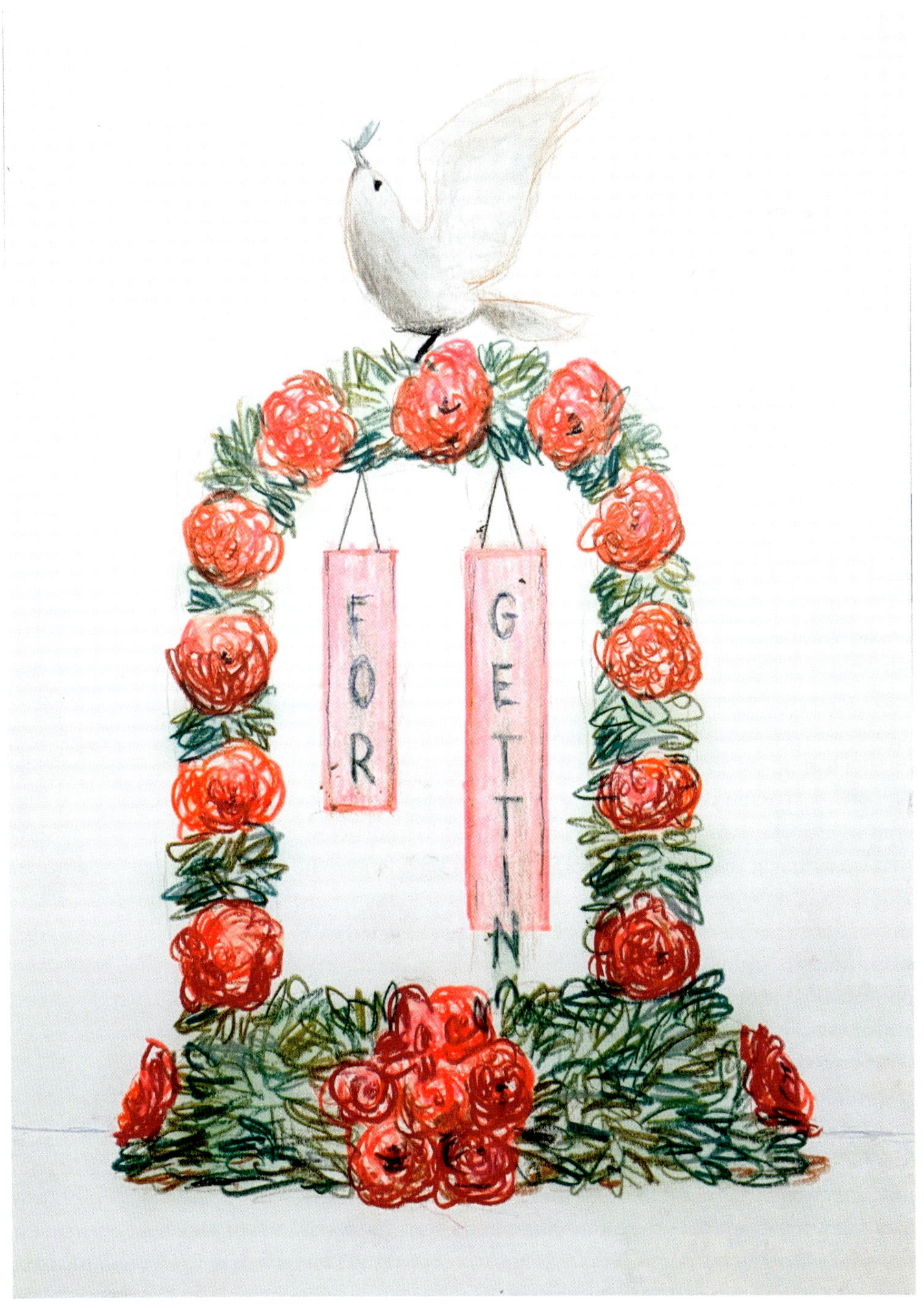
FOR
GETTIN

I CHOSE THE profession of artist for the same reason I chose queerness: escape. I was born in New York City in 1960. Even early on in my life, I knew that I was living a slant from what was expected of me of those beyond my family: I was unathletic, uncomfortable with displays of masculinity, articulate but shy, and drawn to solitude. I had a facility for making things and noted that it was the place where I could not only receive approval, but also where the criteria was my own.

As a teen in the 1970s, I saw the ways that the artworld was a place where I could slip the standard criteria of success and also continue working for the entire span of my life. The artworld that I saw, first at the Bentley School and then at Elisabeth Irwin High School in New York, was not oriented toward commerce. In fact, those people who made a lot of money were treated with suspicion. Artists lived and showed in post-industrial buildings because no one else wanted them. I wanted the life of an artist and always figured that the career would or would not come.

There were no clear guidelines for living that life beyond communication with the people who were living it: other artists. In 1978 I picked my college, Bard, based on the fact that while it was a Liberal Arts College, the arts faculty were practicing artists, not academics. I learned a lot from those artists about pursuing ideas, developing craft, and creating community, but little about providing the material support for that life. Combined with the

Nayland Blake
*Untitled*
2024
12″x9″
Colored pencil on paper
Courtesy of the artist

mixed messages I had gotten from my family about money (it was important, but there wasn't enough of it and I should always be extremely grateful for whatever amount I got) that training left me with little to no long-range planning skills. I had worked from my early teens: paper delivery, babysitting, helping in my mother's shop, on to summer jobs around SoHo in New York City. Getting jobs has never been the problem. Rather, it was the fact that when I got money, I spent it all. I got my first checking account and overdrew it because I didn't bother to balance my account. This was behavior that I would indulge in for years.

I graduated from Bard in 1982 and that summer I moved to Valencia, California, to pursue an MFA at California Institute of the Arts at the suggestion of Nancy Mitchnick, a painter, mentor, and friend who had been my teacher at Bard. In 1984, after two years there, I faced a dilemma: most of my peers were either moving to New York or remaining in LA to pursue their ambitions. I could see that many of my New York friends were grinding away at their lives, trying to have enough money and time to make work, work that was subjected to the arbitrary winds of scrutiny and gallery fashion. I knew two things about my own work: that it was not yet formed enough to withstand those forces, and that I wanted somehow to be out as a queer person in what I made and did. I wanted the work to be a vehicle to explore the complexities of my selfhood and I also didn't feel secure to assert that selfhood in New York's art arena. Perhaps this was another version of my reluctance to engage in competitive machismo. In any event I made the decision that has been the most important in my life and career: I moved to San Francisco, a city I knew very little about, and had only one friend who lived there.

In the early 1980s, San Francisco was no artistic backwater, but it barely registered on New York's radar. It was a city that had three strengths: lots of cheap places to live, a robust nonprofit art scene, and it was the queer capital. In 1984 when I arrived, San Francisco had developed a queer literary and performance culture that had greater complexity and depth than any other place in the United States, a culture that was beginning to feel the worst effects of the AIDS epidemic. That epidemic gave greater urgency to the voices of many artists as well as making it clear that larger societal structures were not going to save us.

My first job in San Francisco was at Just Desserts, a cafe and dessert shop, working the counter. I convinced my manager to allow me to curate monthly art shows on the cafe walls, earning a day off the line and enough money for me to rent space in a studio with three other artists. After a year, I had a show at New Langton Arts, an artist-run nonprofit organization on Folsom Street. After a short while, I was asked to join their artist's board, and was hired as their program coordinator a few years later. I curated shows for them, and participated in nonprofit governance organizations, which allowed me to meet many of the other artists and arts professionals that have sustained my career ever since. I got to function as an advocate for the work from the Bay Area that I thought important, which in turn made people more inclined to look at the work I was making. I continue to believe that artist-run structures allowed me to build my community and to see that community as distinct from a market.

At the end of the 1980s, I had two years of material success, making enough money from my work that I was able to live without a job, move to my own studio, and hire an assistant. Unfortunately, I had gained no additional skills for dealing with money, and so quickly found myself swamped by student debt, credit card debt, and taxes. My largest financial problems came with making money, not with poverty, and it took most of a decade for me to dig myself out of them.

More than anything else, debt has been the greatest obstruction I have faced in my life as an artist. It is the thing that will stop me from working, stop me from speaking to friends, the thing that cuts me off from the sources of joy and pleasure in my work. It was only through years of recovery, therapy, and forbearance on the part of those around me, friends and business associates alike that I was able to come to some semblance of health around debt. The early messages I got from the artists I knew were that "money wasn't important and would somehow work itself out" and that "thinking about finances is antithetical to creative thinking." I've since learned that when I live like that I end up frightened and unable to work. I have to have some sort of clarity about my money situation in order to go into the studio. Getting out of debt was the greatest creative gift I could give myself, and it didn't happen until my early forties.

In 1996, I moved back to New York after fourteen years on the West Coast. I had gallery representation in New York, Los Angeles, and San Francisco, but the market interest in my work had cooled, as had the critical interest. In 1991 I took over a friend's class at the San Francisco Art Institute as a favor and after a while, I found that it was something I had an aptitude for, even though it was a career path that I had decided against years before. Eventually I was teaching multiple courses at a number of institutions in the Bay Area. When I moved to New York, I started to get teaching jobs there: at Parson's, NYU, Bard's master's program, Harvard, and Yale. All of these were single-year contracts as an adjunct. I was essentially a freelancer. Then in 2002, I was approached about the possibility of designing and running a graduate program at the International Center of Photography in partnership with Bard. After doing that job for eighteen years, I have returned to Bard College, now as the co-director of the studio art program I graduated from 40 years ago. I had never thought of myself as an administrator either, but these jobs allow me to continue to work on the vital project of training artists to build an artworld that sustains themselves and their values. I feel like my teaching is a continuation of the cultural lessons I learned in the Bay Area at New Langton. And I feel that everything I do, my teaching, writing, artmaking, curating, and administering is part of the same cultural production.

I am lucky enough that I can do this job in the way that is in keeping with the things that most interest me in making art: the way that individuals can inflect cultural forms, the way that thoughts become objects and thus can be amended or reimagined, the way that creativity provides a refuge for those aslant from dominant culture. The periphery is always more interesting to me than the center, and I'm someone who exists on many borders. But to live on them requires support and encouraging examples. These days I hope to provide one for those coming after me, just as I'm grateful for those who helped me in the past and continue to do so. •

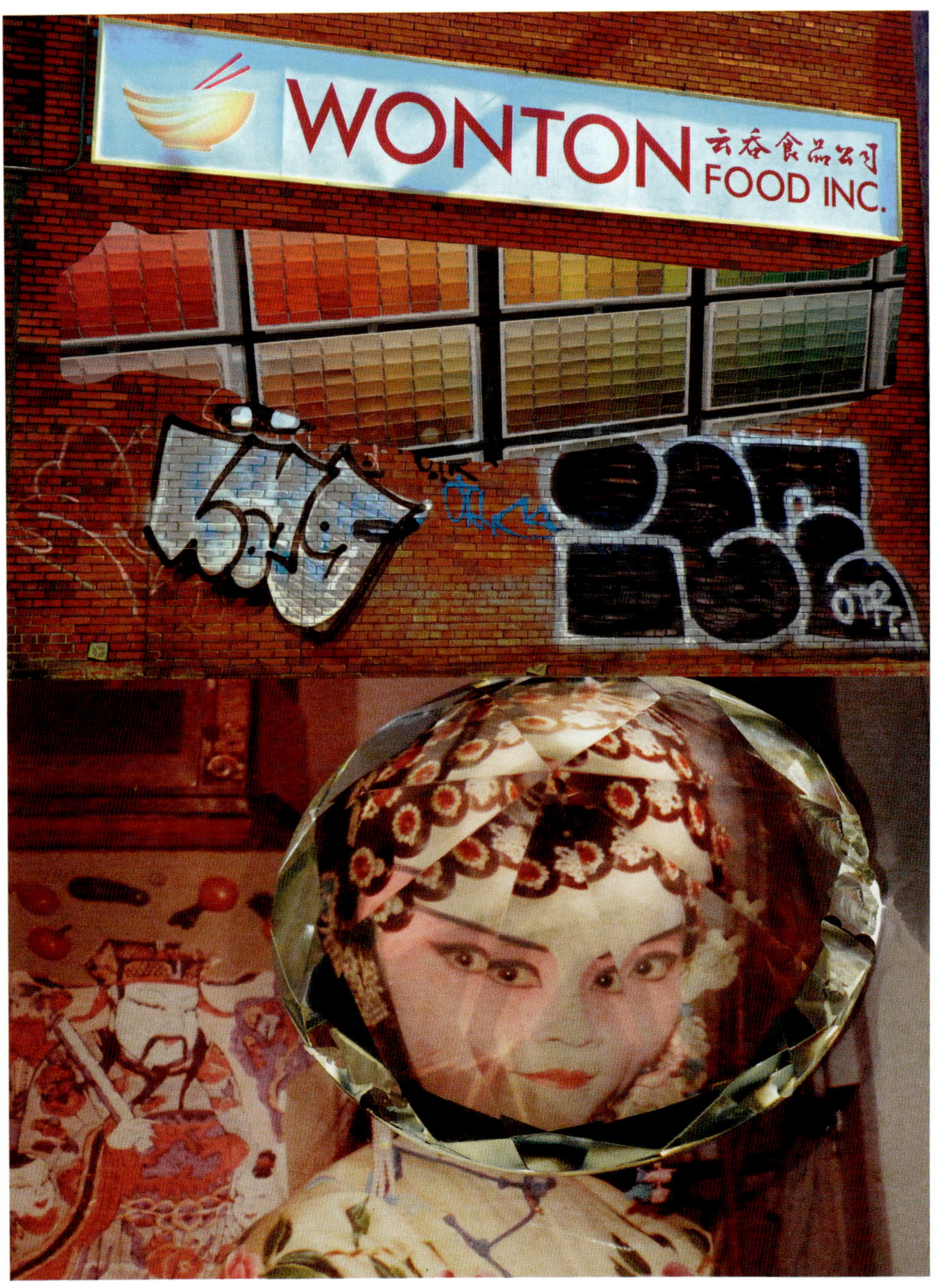
WONTON
云吞食品公司
FOOD INC.

I HAVE EARLY memories of visiting rainy Chinatowns across the country, peering out of our Ford station wagon. Often I'd become more extroverted, so I could be more artistically curious, passionate toward meeting the influences of the magical artists I emulated. My family immigrated from postwar China, moved around a bit, and finally settled in upstate New York. My adventurous artist-dad sought new opportunities even as society was unkind to us—"No to Orientals" was the slogan, as we were labeled--especially difficult during the McCarthy era when seeking housing or jobs. These struggles still recur when I talk to acquaintances, targeting us during the pandemic.

Going back with flashback memories, my adorable mom made Chop Suey sandwiches for school lunches and crafted silk Chinese dresses for my plastic Caucasian dolls! Attending Catholic school early on, "praying" for a heavenly afterlife or applying saints or halos to the compositions was exciting for me as a young artist. Our Western values do dominate when portraying figures and compositions so I needed to unlearn these art practices.

Nina Kuo
*Wonton, Opera Lady*
2022–23
14″x11″
Analog, digital print
Courtesy of the artist

Traveling to foreign countries with my family brought me closer to a realization of class, economic status, and cultural stereotypes. Still feeling frustrated, I closely examined Asian-American diasporic heritages by researching overseas mass media, foreign films, Asian cultural traits, and its pop culture not found in schools or libraries at that time. Ten years later, lecturing and exhibiting in Asia was a huge contrast coming from white suburbia, which made me realize that post-colonial sentiments built our mainstream culture and how we are marginalized through it all.

Luckily in college at State University of New York (SUNY) in Buffalo, I found many dynamic ideas that broke out into new art channels: I hung out with Hallwalls (a nonprofit arts organization based in Buffalo) classmates since we were destined for haphazard lives juggling freelance art careers or temporary jobs. It was essential to move to New York City: the "make it in the art world" mantra.

Experimental color art photographs started to be a big deal. I put aside painting, yet I was always attracted to the floating, torn-up montages of urban landscapes made possible by abstracting painted compositions. For decades, in cold months or spending weeks in hot smelly darkrooms, I'd return to making painted works in my cheap apartment, commonly moving around to save on rent. I'd recycle found materials and use them for props, in photographic or 2-D works, etc. It was so rewarding to reuse materials and I am ecstatic when they are reinvented. As my work revealed created built-up surfaces like close-up dot matrices found in color negatives, I envisioned mimicked upstate snow days—my favorite natural phenomenon. I even made videos of these colored dots. I wanted to be "Dot" the comic book character. I also loved playing make-believe theater with my artsy sister and adding colored filters with flashlights, which was delightful.

Thereby, I was destined to become a visual artist. Ultimately to express my independent self-made identity overcoming my love-hate sense of old world expectations. I started attending feminist groups: Judy Chicago workshop and others as an undergraduate gave me insight to be a totally aligned feminist. I adopted feminist critical theories as my art quest expanded and would take much planning. I had few real supportive colleagues then as full-time job challenges became real and the artworld demanded more artistic skills from us single POC women. For decades East Coast Asian-American Art was undefined to art historians or mainstream artworld gurus. Additional exposure to these aesthetics needed to be prepared and researched. Pioneer POC art movements seemed progressive. Transforming marginalized communities' new leaders and ethnic groups created shared bonds of camaraderie. Our ad-hoc and experimentally avant-garde policies proved our validity as artists.

Luckily being hired as a salaried Comprehensive Employment Training Act (CETA) artist meant exposure to diverse, multi-ethnic artists, writers, musicians, etc. That network offered citywide collaborations and placed me early at the Basement Workshop (an Asian American cultural center), which focused on ad-hoc arts skills and self-taught administrative tasks.

Through this camaraderie, the CETA documentation unit and colleagues Dawoud Bey, Danny Dawson, and others commissioned my works. It epitomized how cool multiculturalists related to each other. Other artists and myself pressed onwards, challenging existing art practices. We broke out completely, playing by our own free rules—depicting the growing influence of visual artists, writers, and mentors who challenged artworld tactics through alternative art spaces, which became explosive as the years spun by.

Meanwhile, my color "Contrapted" series was selected in JAM Gallery's group exhibition in 1978 and accepted for an iconic 1982 *Black Currents* journal, which Janet Henry boldly curated. Then after some lean years, I met my partner, Lorin Roser, who gave me close ties to experimental architectural and multimedia arts. Who knew we would go onto shared passions of free-spirited lifestyles and raw downtown art scenes! In order to survive, we had freelance administrative, teaching, or gallery gigs, ultimately giving us free time to make weird art.

In the same circle of transplanted artists and new émigrés, the art scene in New York City was budding with new vigor. The next wave of artist-run galleries supported this influx of artists! No wonder avant-garde and multicultural art spaces with artist curators sprouted out to the Bronx like En Foco, and Fred Wilson's restored Longwood Art Gallery in 1987 where I exhibited in the group show *Room with a View*. It was upbeat as uptown spaces arrived with downtown popularity.

As numerous art spaces brought on radical changes in the art world, there were ups and downs. Most significantly I met dynamo Marcia Tucker. For her *Bad Girls* 1994 group show, I composed myself with two Asian American women wearing Chinese garb, which I titled *Calendar Girls.* Our stereotyped women's jobs were listed in the wall label text (the unrelated occupations for women revealed a sense of our disjointed professional lives), for example: waitress, babysitter, paralegal, editor, weather girl, teacher, administrator, designer, model maker, etc. Truly a career mish-mosh that most women must accept in order to make ends meet. There was little glamour in that statement.

In continuing Asian American Pacific Islander (AAPI) art, I organized the first Asian-American artist registry and organized a panel with critic and writer Lucy Lippard and art leaders. The art public witnessed how AAPI art had mileage and my confidence and reputation soared. I realized linking savvy POC artists was vital in becoming more publicly accepted and thus deserving of art funding. Feminists I knew, such as Howardena Pindell, Camille Billops, etc., urged us to unite by joining activists' groups such as Heresies, Pests, etc., (Godzilla came later on and there's even a book about its legacy). Because there are more internationally connected art circles, this catalyst engaged a shared transformation of cultural equality.

In the early 1980s, I witnessed and met "one-year performance artist" Tehching Hsieh, who gave me humility and higher determination to life balances and how one's artistic philosophy comes from freeing oneself from the complexities of bureaucracies or art rules. Comparing my artistic practice with a long time span was the proper presentation of one's cultural identity. We would share tips on renovating and how to master being minimal and frugal.

I now can see ghosts along the way in this period of art movements: hierarchies, art markets, and how a balanced representation brought on new connections for galleries and public art. The many expectations and conformity had to be reinvented by supporting alternative art spaces and independent thinkers. We witnessed early artists and administrators transforming geopolitical cultural movements. Since Thelma Golden, Kellie Jones, and Lydia Yee curated me in group shows, I had to take bigger risks in art experimentation during down years.

Job hopping—in museums, schools, galleries, editorial and fashion companies, even making soft models for Gaetano Pesce or Maggie Cheung film shoots—was getting tiresome. I ventured into art therapy, a demanding yet stable career path. I had the "on the job" training as it prepared me for many roles. I witnessed ongoing mental challenges and emotional problems that existed in many levels of society. The clinical staff emphasized an atmosphere built on trust and caring teamwork.

After work hours, I created multicultural workshops, concerts with my contacts and even helped curate art shows for disadvantaged people. These influences brought together plans to make tributes to Steve Cannon, Ntozake Shange, etc., even making artist books and 3-D works. That is how making art became for me: a backdrop for pursuing a more spirited life that was rewarding and challenging for years. When making a difference as an arts leader, these roles gave me a deeper sense of emotional worth and mutual intellectual expressiveness.

Today's high-tech world is a multifaceted challenge, to give up simple technical tasks while adapting creative, zany, satiric art projects. It's hard to focus on how low technology will serve us versus robotic, high-tech chores. Usually I create a lot of artwork, never destined to be seen, or I build bodies of thematic works as they become totally intimate the longer I work on them. These long-term projects make me observe my subject matter, which is often physically demanding. As I age, I see health and wellness making a huge difference to my artistic practice. I learned about Moxibustion on early trips to Asia. While traveling or going to art residencies, it offered relief for sore muscles and satisfaction for stress relief so I made fast friends. These rare moments are a shared meditation—like in acupuncture as nature's ability to heal is holistic and vital. There's a constant stress level, and reassurance is needed to reinforce our modern psyche.

I felt we must interpret how artists are trained to be multifaceted, good at multitasking, yet multicultural while trying to be in the metaverse! I feel an urgency when I work due to the COVID-19 virus and recent pandemic. We need to make up for lost time. Having my work shown in current exhibitions is truly inspiring and encapsulates many early multimedia aesthetics, crossovers of minds and genres, which present a union of minds where old and new acquaintances are offered new insights. Hopefully our legacies will be restored and our multicultural inclusion regains importance.

Since there is no orderly system in my daily work, I must constantly stay on top of it all. It can be digital editing, shoots, archiving or actual art processes in the making. Through some dealers, and fairs, I get the roller coaster of experiences. It is unpredictable what curators are looking for but I keep attentive and respond to different requests over the years. I zig zag ideas for requested thematic works. Whether addressing global warming that depict floods, polluted bamboo showing devastation—it's all demanding. Learning tech skills constantly usurps my time while the constant push and pull between different media  is exciting.

Geographically, the outer boroughs of New York City have become more ethnic, offering more BIPOC collaborators. Dancers, performance artists, etc., are my subjects. I plug into doing experimental collaborations with my partner: informal performance videos or with public projected stills. Recently I addressed AAPI racist attacks with handmade posters and prepared a cinematic montage mural in 2022 addressing domestic violence, which became a neighborhood solution for its working-class citizens. I have a strong belief in preserving cultural lore and histories as I look at operas, ethnic dress, mores in folk art, etc.

It's fantastic to create digital art, which has opened arenas in new media as the digital art travels on its own trajectory especially for collaborative international online worlds. I aim to solve the mind's life investigations in an honest, just manner with new media technologies as a starting point.

With mixed medias or video technologies, my simple aim of capturing new idioms of refuge is how I survived being isolated in the studio. I can openly memorialize expressive dreams and channel sensual, ritualistic expressions that free me from stereotypes or bondage as I make homages to archaeological clay figures. “Let’s Move the Crowd,” a phrase from rallies and mass media, invented spiritual, cultural, and mental icons of our shared persona. It is positive for me to combat today’s issues that affect many people, especially in post-pandemic times, with expressive messages going forward. ●

# PATTI WARASHINA

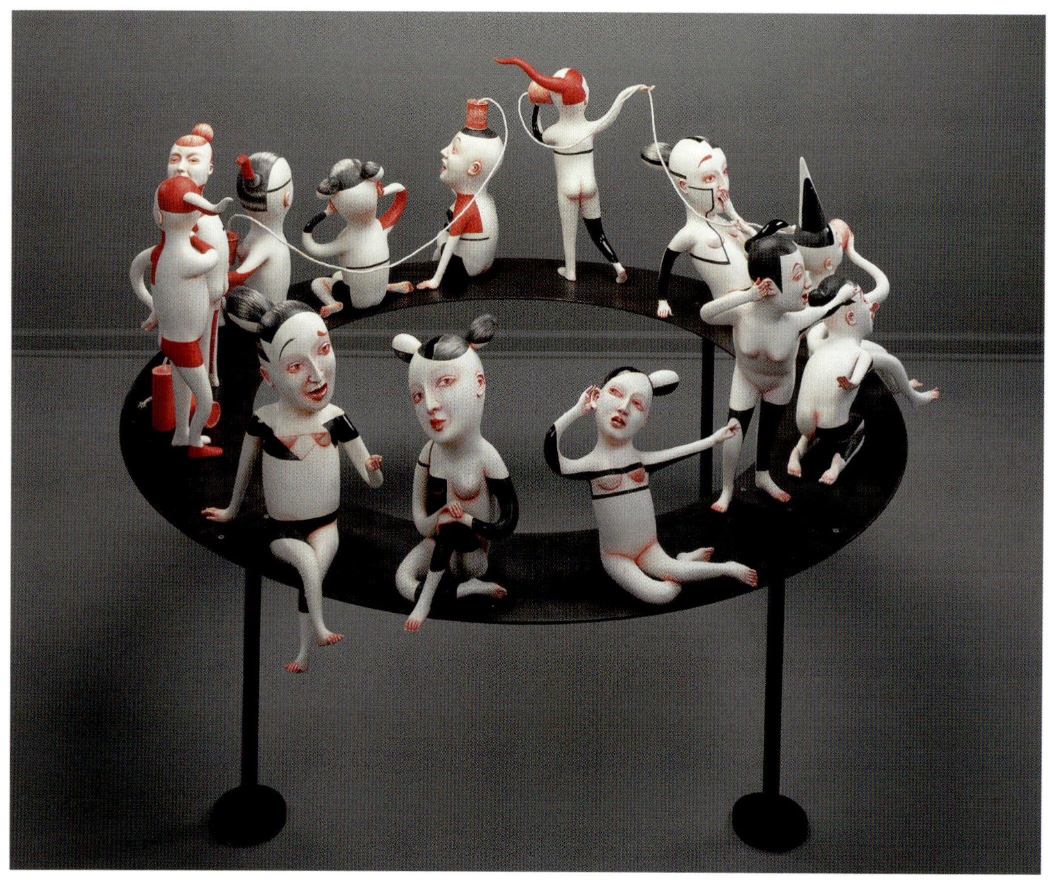

Patti Warashina
*Gossipmongers*
2010
25″x84″x84″ (24″ stand)
Low-fire clay, underglaze, glaze, mixed media, steel
Courtesy of the artist
Photography by Rob Vinnedge

I OFTEN THINK about what my life might have been had I not discovered art in my undergraduate years in college. God saved society when I decided *not* to become a dental hygienist or medical technologist, which was my intended purpose in going to college.

Looking back over the past 50 years of being a professional artist, my thoughts go back to how difficult and stressful it was during my early career being a single mom, raising a family, and teaching, all at the same time. That era stands out most vividly in my memory.

In my youth growing up in Spokane, Washington, during the 1940s, 1950s, and early 1960s, my Japanese-American parents were vigilant in encouraging their children to get an academic education with their financial support. They wanted the best for the future of their children, to be self-sufficient, since they had endured "trying" lives through the "war." I knew early on that I would be going to the coastal city of Seattle for college, as there was a large Asian community for support. Spokane, though a sizable "inland" city from Seattle, had a much smaller Japanese community. At that time, the city of Spokane was a railroad center and lacked the visual culture and arts found in coastal cities such as San Francisco, Los Angeles, and Seattle.

Being an artist was the furthest profession from my mind when I started at the University of Washington in 1958. Prior to college, I had been raised to believe that academic studies were integral to finding a future career. As a science major, I took a required "elective" course in beginning drawing. This class captured my imagination, and it was only a matter of time before I started taking more art classes. Needless to say, I never left. My beginning ceramic class was very compelling. I found the "feel" and the challenge of manipulating the clay totally addictive and absorbing. It is the sensuous nature of the clay that has kept my focus on this material for the better part of my life. I indulged my fascination for this material by "sneaking" and hiding myself during "off hours" in the ceramic studio, and oftentimes being reported to the campus police. After a while, the "office" and the campus police gave up, disregarded the reports, and figured that I would be an asset in guarding the ceramic studio during "off" hours. There was a point in time when I did not know what an "artist" was. It wasn't until much later that I realized that an "artist" was someone who was driven to work in the studio, much like the need to eat and sleep.

That early "basic training" revealed the technical difficulties in building and firing clay, but it was also a time to concentrate on how to overcome or "go around" those unending annoyances as one advances to the next idea or stage of work. It has been a cumulative learning curve over the years, and because of the challenging "nature of the beast," I've always felt, as a clay artist, that you had to be either focused . . . or a blithering masochist . . . because the kiln and the material have the final "say." The work of Peter Voulkos, Robert Arneson, Robert Sperry, and other early experimental clay artists on the West Coast brought new excitement to me. Clay, as a medium of personal expression, became more relevant, especially when the Funk Movement on the West Coast exposed clay to the world as a viable, legitimate medium for contemporary artistic expression.

My generous widowed mother helped me financially through art school, as she said that if I had found something I truly loved to do that I "would do well in it," and she supported me wholeheartedly. In 1962, my first job and experience in teaching was as a teacher's assistant at the University of Washington in graduate school, when the Director of the School of Art Boyer Gonzales came to my studio and told me about teaching a design class.

It was the first time I realized that teaching in college was a possibility, and a possible way to support my own art.

At the end of graduate school, I married fellow graduate student Fred Bauer in 1964 before moving to the Midwest for teaching positions. I subsequently had two daughters while teaching in the Midwest for four years. My first year of teaching was at Wisconsin State University, Platteville. The next three years we lived in Ann Arbor, Michigan, where I taught at Eastern Michigan University in Ypsilanti. Being in the Midwest, I was able to travel and meet a lot of other Midwest and East Coast artists. We returned to Seattle in 1968 where I continued teaching at Cornish College of the Arts and the University of Washington night school, which later became a full-time position after my divorce in 1969.

My early clay studios were always in the basements of my houses, and the hot ceramic kilns kept safely in the garage. This arrangement of working in the home allowed the children to be in close proximity, and I could work late into the night after they'd gone to bed. After my divorce, working in the studio became therapeutic, but it was also necessary to retain a position at a research university which required teaching, working in the studio, traveling for lectures, and exhibiting. It was a crazy time, raising two small children under these circumstances. I recall a long list of babysitters in those early years that I often had to prevail upon to take up the slack. I am fortunate that I have a genetic flaw that allows me to keep late hours, and wake up early to get on with the day's work without feeling "totally out of it." I was also fortunate that my two daughters accepted and understood that I had to work in the studio to survive, and accepted the fact that I would not be like the typical "Leave it to Beaver" mother in the 1960s and could not be home to greet them with milk and cookies. It was imperative that they had to help me by getting home on time, being responsible and well behaved. After "Saturday clean-ups," the three of us would sit on the stairway in our home and have "confessions," sharing any complaints they had about me during the past week. In their child-like voices they would tell me the issues they had with my parenting. I, in turn, would equally tell them what bothered me about their behavior during the week!!! Weekly confession time, I think, was cathartic for the three of us, and kept us in communication. I also used to tell them that after 8:30 p.m. was my time to work in the studio, sometimes till 2:00 or 3:00 a.m. in the morning. Our family motto during those difficult years was, "YOU'RE ON YOUR OWN."

An eye-opening episode during that busy time of balancing the job of being an exhibiting artist, teacher, and mother was when a preschool mother, Paula Grey, invited my two daughters to stay overnight on a weekend for a "playdate" with her daughter. When my daughters arrived home the next morning, my daughter Lisa said to me, "Mommy, you AREN'T supposed to make toast like you do!" I looked at her quizzically, and said, "What do you mean?" Lisa responded, "I told Mrs. Grey that you are supposed to take the toast to the sink and SCRAPE IT!!!!!" I looked at her, mortified, as I would be seeing Paula Grey at preschool the coming week. After about seven years, I remarried to a wonderful ceramic artist, Robert Sperry, who helped co-parent with me, and didn't burn the toast. We were married for about 21 years before he sadly passed away in 1998.

After 30 years of teaching, I retired from the University of Washington in 1995. I have been able to exhibit and work in my studio consistently over the past 50 years, as it was not only a necessity for teaching, but I found working in my studio was "like going to a shrink," with no appointment necessary! Initially, while young, work was submitted to competitive shows, and over time, exposure of my work brought it to the attention of other artists, collectors, and galleries. It is fortunate, for me and those close to me, that I was able to find a compelling interest in my life, which continues to this day to be evolving and challenging. Whether it is a "hit or a miss," trying to envision a visual image in my mind's eye, and hoping to see it come to "life," still continues to absorb me!! In a nutshell, I think my curious nature and love of "problem solving" is what continues to lure me to the studio. I see my work as a visual diary and can look back at my work and see what was happening during my own life. Over the years, after honing my skills in clay, I have found that it not only brings on more problems and images to resolve, but expands the possibilities of more ideas to explore. It seems endless and open-ended, and looking back over the years, never boring. My only regret is that time is going by so rapidly, and it is frustrating not to be able to lengthen the span of the day!

This may sound maudlin, but looking back over time, I couldn't have asked for a more fulfilling life than being an artist, with such wonderful and interesting friends, and people from all walks of life that I met through my travels, teaching, family, my studio work, and just general living. It has also kept me out of a mental institution!! ●

PRINCESS SIMPSON RASHID

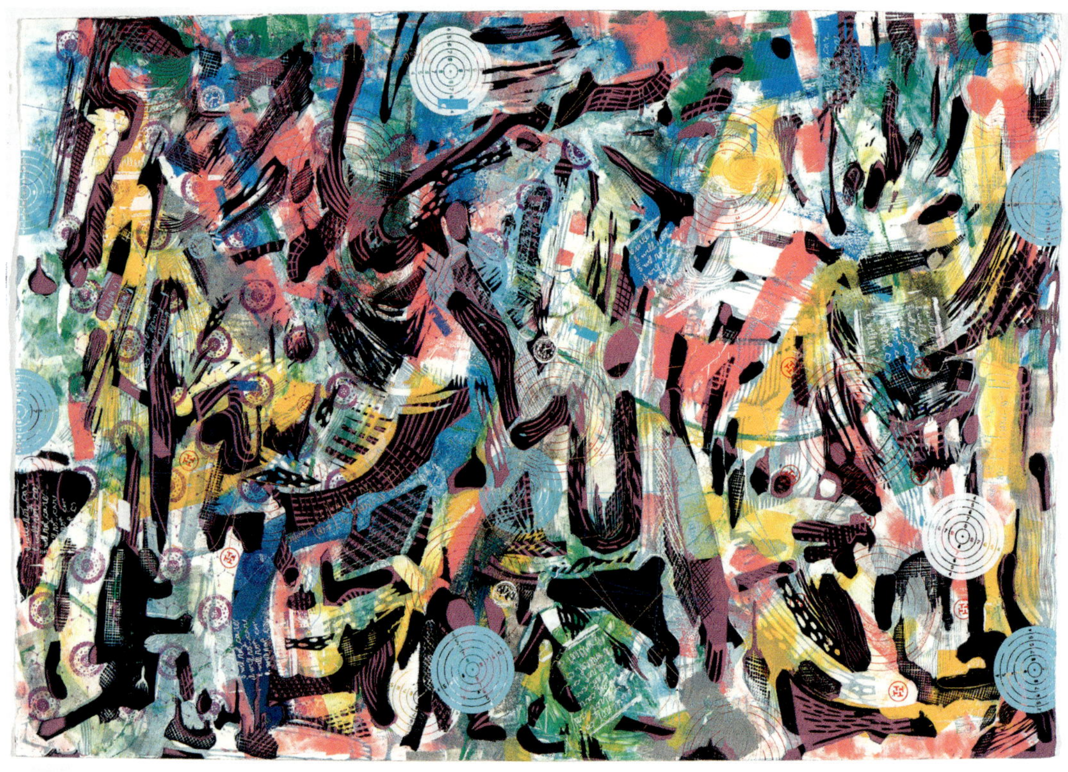

Princess Simpson Rashid
*Destruction of the Temple*
2020
36″x54″
Monoprint
Courtesy of the artist
Photography by Sean Kelly
Conway

*HOW DID I get here?* I wanted a family *and* a career. When I graduated college in 1995, this sentiment was top of mind. Which was weird because as an undergraduate physics student at Georgia State University in Atlanta, I hadn't thought much about having a family at all.

Like most young people, I struggled with identity, who I would be. Upon graduation, another recession hit the country and job prospects were dim. The internet was still young and information wasn't as easily obtainable as it is now. After years of stellar service, my father was embroiled in a crisis at his job and my parents' marriage was struggling. I was becoming disillusioned by everything I trusted.

Early on, while working on my degree, I received a lot of support, but when my program advisors heard I was getting married they seemed to drop their interest in supporting my career as a scientist and/or scholar. Advisement ceased. It felt like now I was seen as a wasted commodity.

At the time, I was only sure about one thing. I wanted to marry my fiancé. He was my guy, but what I didn't understand at the time was that he was already married to the Navy which would eventually pose a problem for me.

Thanks to my mother, I had a Renaissance-style upbringing when we lived in Plainfield, New Jersey, in the late 1970s through the 1980s. In addition to attending public school, she provided me with a structured home regimen and I was compliant.

My time was occupied with music and ballet lessons, reading quotas, repetition exercises, and science experiments. I didn't understand it when I was kid, but she was grooming me to be a life-long learner driven by my curiosities.

In addition, my aunt and her husband, Earnestine Rainey and James Huff, were working artists. In 1972, the year I was born, they founded Huff Art Studio in Winston-Salem, North Carolina, and started building a community-driven art practice. They were the first real artists I knew and were very generous, giving me insights about how to build and maintain a collector base.

Over the course of four decades, they raised a family, were activists in their community and exhibited nationally and internationally. They showed me that making a living as artists was not only possible but sustainable.

From 1998 to 2000, I studied painting, printmaking and sculpture at the Escuela de Artes Plásticas y Diseño de Puerto Rico in Old San Juan, Puerto Rico. I remember one of my professors, Zilia Sánchez, telling me, as a young married female art student, to keep my own name as I build my career. Because of her, I make it a point to include my maiden name in all my formal art documentation. She impressed upon me the validity and need to protect the integrity of my individual identity, especially as a woman and as an artist.

In 2018, it was a great encouragement to me when I came across her work *Untitled* from the series *Erotic Topography* at The Pérez Art Museum Miami (PAMM) during Art Basel. The abstract and conceptual nature of her work continue to inform my own.

Early on in my career, I wondered if it was possible to be a successful artist and mother. The sculptor and printmaker, Elizabeth Catlett, provided me with an excellent example of both. In addition to being a wife and mother of three children, she continued to be an activist and prolific artist.

In 2003, I got a chance to meet her at a retrospective lecture at the Telfair Museum of Art in Savannah, Georgia. I remember, with one of her adult sons hovering protectively in the wings, she shared slides of her different bodies of work that spanned decades. She expressed how she couldn't wait to get back home to Mexico to carve a huge eight-foot chunk of African mahogany she'd ordered.

To me, that was awesome. In her late 80s, she had the passion to continue making. She worked with her whole body in such a physical way. Wood carving demanded it. Her example was so instructive to me. It was a seed I kept to fuel the artistic life I wanted to build.

I had my first child in 2000 and the second in 2008. Both pregnancies had many complications but each had their standouts. The day I received news that my dear grandfather had passed, the first baby I carried went into distress. My doctor informed me that I was experiencing preterm labor and I would have to go on full bed rest for the last three months of the pregnancy. So, it seemed the first baby was determined to come out too early. Eight years later, the second baby tried to stay in too long and I developed a condition called PUPPP, pruritic urticarial papules and plaques of pregnancy. It is a horrible itchy rash that appears in stretch marks of the stomach and other parts during late term. Fortunately, despite these and other complications, both my girls were born healthy.

In the early days, I didn't have a studio outside my home. I made time to paint by working when everyone else went to bed. Nine p.m. to 2:00 a.m. was my art-making time. But as I matured as an artist, I realized having a studio separate from my home was important for me. And whenever able, I would secure one, despite having to move frequently due to the demands of being part of a Navy family.

The most impactful studio location I've had to date is my current one, at CoRK Arts District (CoRK) in Jacksonville, FL. CoRK is an 800,000+ square feet warehouse complex that is home to close to 70 artists and related businesses. Being a resident artist there has provided me with tremendous creative camaraderie and opportunities for fruitful collaboration. It is a sanctuary where I can work for uninterrupted blocks of time.

However, shortly after I secured a studio space at CoRK, in 2014, I was diagnosed with Stage 2 breast cancer. I had a mastectomy and underwent chemotherapy and immunotherapy. It was a tough time. I still suffer from side effects, like neuropathy, lymphedema, chronic pain, and fatigue. My last chemotherapy session was in 2016. I was 42 when diagnosed. Now, I'm 52 as I write this. I lost a decade to treatment and recovery. But I did gain a few things.

In my fight with breast cancer, I attribute my years of training as a competitive fencer, which I started back in college, with giving me the fortitude to not give up. How to fight, accepting small wins and losses with the big ones, and most importantly, how to push through pain were some of the things I learned from competitive fencing.

Ironically, the money I made through fencing often supplemented my art practice—everything from sales of fencing art, teaching classes, and giving private lessons to running a fencing club as the head coach.

Another thing that got me through treatment was writing. Poetry. Bad poetry. But eventually, I found a local writing coach, Lynn Skapyak Harlin, and started to improve. I'm currently working on my first poetry collection. I'm beginning to get published in literary journals and have been asked to perform and read at literary festivals. Building my reputation as a writer is important to me. It complements the career I've built in the visual arts.

After multiple surgeries and chemotherapy, I felt like the mythical phoenix rising from the ashes of who I used to be. The woman in the mirror was now so different in appearance and temperament. My art needed to change too. The chaos of illness sent me on a hunt for pattern, meaning, and order.

In 2016, while still in active treatment, I was commissioned to create a suite of monotypes for an exhibit at the Cummer Museum of Art & Gardens in Jacksonville, Florida, entitled *Lift: Contemporary Expressions of the African American Experience.* That project was a lifeline for me. It was a physical and mental challenge because of chemo-fatigue and peripheral neuropathy affecting my hands and feet. But despite the discomfort, my spirit was encouraged. I believed the work mattered.

In the spring of 2020, the COVID-19 pandemic and economic shutdown hit hard and again things went a little dark.

Artist opportunities dried up. Temporarily, I had to move out of my studio and work strictly from home.

I think this period helped me become even more introspective. I went through tons of my neglected old sketchbooks and journals. I started to want to show evidence of mark-making in my art, no longer embarrassed by my known chicken scratch. I saw it as evidence of my humanity. The more I turned inward the more confident in myself I became.

Being stuck at home gave me another special gift. I noticed birds courting, butterflies and bees flying about, and squirrels playing in my backyard. All things I hardly paid attention to when the world was normal before the pandemic.

By the fall, some institutions were cautiously opening up and I was invited to serve as the artist in residence at Trident Editions, a print atelier and subsidiary of Florida State College of Jacksonville (FSCJ). To be invited to work with a master printmaker was a dream. So when Patrick Miko of Trident Editions extended the invitation, I was honored. Despite the constraints of the pandemic, we generated a large body of work—a suite of eleven large format monoprints (36 × 54 inches) and 28 smaller prints of various sizes on handmade paper.

This project stretched my thinking in terms of scale, layering, and the power of masterful collaboration. I am a stronger printmaker because of the experience and the work we produced. All the little observations I'd made during the shutdown incubated, so when I began work on this new series, I had plenty of ideas and raw material to mine.

In 2021, I completed another artist residency in Jacksonville. This time at the Museum of Science & History (MOSH). I created a four-panel mural called the *Wonder Wall*. It has been installed as the signature piece in their "creation station." The work synthesized my research and ideas about the relationship between neuroscience, visual perception, and creativity. My design process placed special emphasis on the "doodle" and "squiggle" as important exploratory elements for idea generation, memory encoding and recall. After being sick, memory became something I wanted to explore.

Both the pandemic and my cancer experience made me take stock of my life. I searched for meaning and substance, which led me to compose abstractions that were more socially and politically conscious. But also now I attempt to embed spaces for play and curiosity in the work when possible.

Recently, I've started an urban sketching practice in order to document my environment, one sketch at a time. It's a commitment to learn how to see. I journal and write to learn what I think. Writing and sketching enhances my art practice. They keep the spark alive in me as I continue to build my artistic life, brick by brick. •

# RANU MUKHERJEE

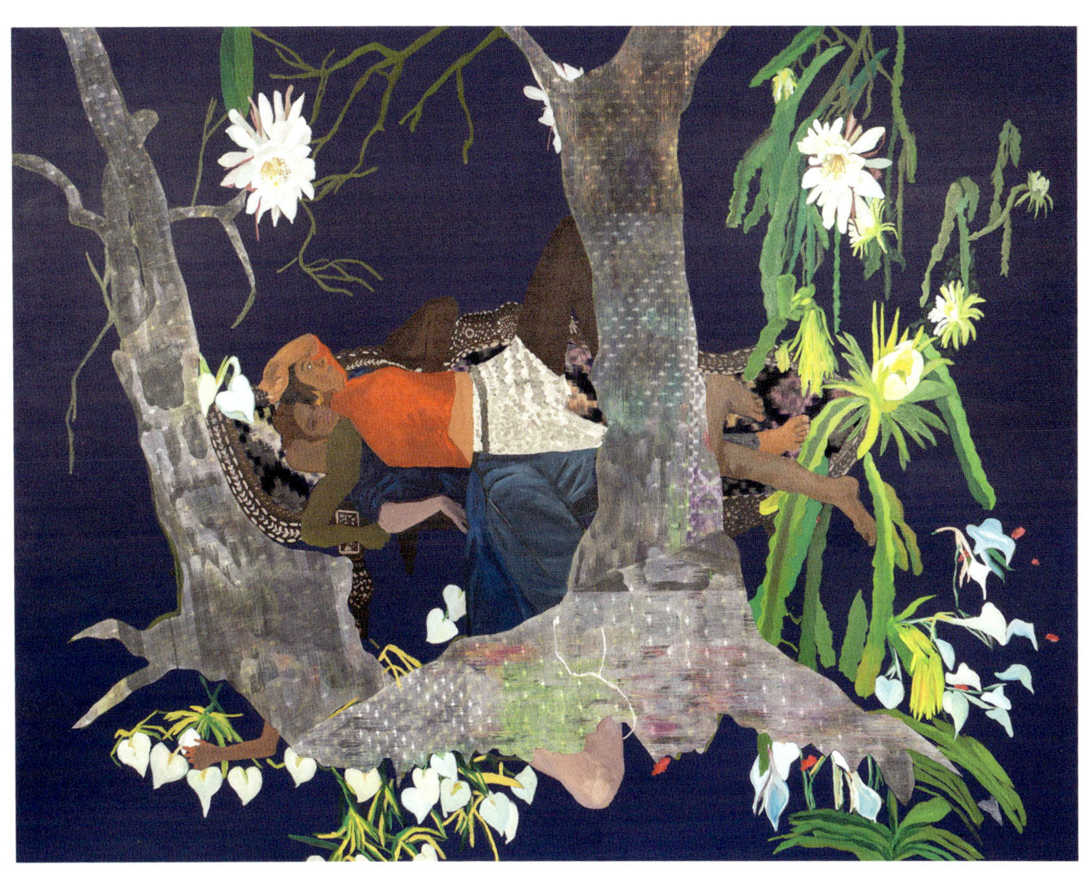

As with most families, mine included people who made things. They were Italian-Americans who carved gravestones and made crochet doll clothes. My German-American grandfather worked in a foundry and sent me precious drawings that he made with a ballpoint pen. My father, Sunirmal Mukherjee, fled from Dhaka with his family to settle in Kolkata in the 1940s in the lead up to the end of British rule and partition of India. I imagine him growing up surrounded by the legacies of Gandhi, Tagore, and the revolutionary school Santiniketan. After immigrating to the United States in the early 1960s, he was killed in an accident in Gilroy, California, not far from San Francisco where I currently live. I was 18 months old.

I don't really consider my art to be primarily about self-expression, but the elements of my father's culture that were left in the house (such as a book of mythological prints and a pile of sari cloth given to my mother for when we moved back to India), have become major references and materials in my work. My fascination with non-linear time and speculative fiction probably emerged from this rupture, and the consciousness of a parallel life I would have led had he not been killed.

Growing up as a misrecognized, mixed-race person in a white suburb was also a significant experience in terms of navigating otherness and the demand for legibility that is served up to people of color in the United States. Octavia Butler's writing

Ranu Mukherjee
*Restless Moon*
2023
60″x84″
Pigment, ink, crystalina, and UV inkjet print on silk and cotton sari fabric and cotton ikat on linen
Courtesy of Gallery Wendi Norris
Photography by Scott Saraceno Photography

showed me early on that it was possible to make work that was complex, critical, and joyful in response to these conditions.

I attended public schools from kindergarten through high school in my hometown of Newton, Massachusetts. I had no idea that being an artist was a thing that living people did until my junior year when I met a representative from Massachusetts College of Art at the college fair in my high school cafeteria. I was drawn to her difference and ended up deciding, in a totally intuitive way, to follow this attraction.

I am often surprised by the things I find myself doing as an artist; this is one of the gifts of our occupation. Most of the artists I know have taken winding pathways. I am well into the second major chapter of my art life.

From 1994–2003, I worked almost exclusively as part of the collective-as-avatar called "0rphan Drift." I co-created this formation in London in 1994 with three other artists, Susanne Karakashian, Maggie Mer Roberts, and Erle Stenberg, shortly after I completed my MA in Painting at the Royal College of Art (RCA) (1991). I had managed to get two degrees without going into debt, starting with a BFA in Painting with a minor in filmmaking from the Massachusetts College of Art (Mass Art) (1988). Tuition at Mass Art was $600 per semester then and the RCA gave me a scholarship that covered a year of tuition. Their rate for international students was lower than most schools in the United States, so despite the fact that London was an expensive place to live, I was able to graduate and enjoy the privilege of being a broke experimental artist for a few years.

"Professional practice" courses did not really exist then. I knew I was in the long game and assumed it would take time to develop work that had significance. Some artists had families that could buy them a studio when they graduated and EU citizens could collect unemployment. I was in neither position after finishing my MA, so I got a job at the Literary Review Club in SoHo, London, making soup, serving pork pies, and pouring a lot of scotch. I was also fortunate to be offered a part-time teaching position in visual arts at Goldsmiths College by my graduate advisor Sam Fisher in the renowned BFA program that several of the Young British Artists (YBAs) had graduated from. I had not seriously considered teaching but this opened the way for what is now a 27-year occupation running alongside my studio work.

From 1992–95, A few of us lived in a huge shared house on Agar Grove in Camden. I remember piling around a gas heater in the cold foggy winters in a funky basement living room that had glass doors out to an overgrown backyard. There was a weird little kitchenette and we used to drink PG Tips with milk in pint glasses. We staged an exhibition there, using all of the rooms, and got favorable reviews for it. The journalists paid attention to artist-led cultural production that was abundant in London at that time. There was a ghost of a woman who had been abused in her life in the house. Some of us could hear her scream at night. The artist Steve Claydon, who also lived there, made a piece that looked like a police cordon in the backyard. The neighbors came around asking if the body buried there had been found. They showed us marks in the ceiling they said were from brass knuckles.

0rphan Drift worked across the cultural spheres of contemporary art, electronic music, renegade academia, and experimental film and my art life was characterized by an anarchic DIY ethos, shared resources, cyberpunk and collective production. We played with models that challenged individual authorship and binary divisions between critical thinking and pop culture. I think working in London in the early nineties, as artists coming up after the Young British Art movement, had something to do with choosing to work this way. I felt awkward and out of place in the art scene and ran in the opposite direction from the "artist as celebrity" that seemed very prominent at the time. I also didn't feel aligned with the minimal aesthetics of European conceptualism. We were instead inspired by groundbreaking polyrhythmic electronic music, particularly the Jungle nights at the Paradise Club in Islington and the ethos of white label production.

We installed immersive installations that involved sleeping in galleries for days. We played VJ gigs at underground music nights, in squats, and under the archways that are now the new Kings Cross. We made performance lectures and collaborated with other makers and thinkers—notably the group called BANK, the Cybernetic Culture Research Unit, Kodwo Eshun, Kode9 and the Spaceape, and the founders of Virtual Futures, Otto Imken and Dan O'Hara. I also worked and traveled with John Cussans, my partner at the time. With the onset of the internet age, I dreamed of a nomadic lifestyle. In 1995 I bought my first laptop and we went to Mexico for 6 months. Like many aspects of that cultural moment, nomadic life eventually became almost required of artists.

Some people called 0rphan Drift a cult because we described our work as a signal and didn't use our individual names. Interviewers often resorted to commenting on our dyed hair or reptilian pets. Our work exemplified feminist practice aligned with Donna Haraway's "A Cyborg Manifesto." But our lifestyle was physically exhausting. I started doing yoga in the year 1999, after our project Syzygy, a complex grant funded project at Beaconsfield Arts in London. That was a watershed moment. I began to pay more attention to my health and environment, to cultivate presence in a different way. After that, we all began to drift again.

»

I am indebted to that experience in many ways, to the London of the 1990s, to an immersive collectivity, to the visionary people I was surrounded by who saw the world changing and wanted to play a part in making something new. Many of them are still very close friends and I see the imprint of that time in the work they do today. The 1990s work of 0rphan Drift is a slice of that history. Artist and friend Maggie Roberts and I continue working together, across continents. The current iteration of 0rphan Drift is again in dialogue with the context of rapid technological development, questioning the presence of artificial intelligence in current narratives of futurity within a global environmental crisis.

In 2006 I gave birth to triplets, Simone, Sunil, and Lelio, who are now 18 years old (at the time of writing). I had moved to San Francisco in 2003 to be with their father Mike Maurillo, a sound designer who has made many of the scores to my films. Mike was my brother David's college roommate at UC Berkeley and we had fallen in love just after 9/11. I was visiting San Francisco from London to decide if I wanted to move here, staying in David's rent-controlled apartment in the Mission District, a block from Mike's rent-controlled apartment. The morning of September 11th, David came into my room and said, "Sis. You better get up, a plane just hit the World Trade Center." A little while later Mike came over because his TV was broken. He is from Brooklyn and had two siblings working near the towers when they fell.

The few years after I moved to San Francisco, between 2003 and 2009, were a major period of transition that in some ways felt like starting all over again. After working under a different name, on a different continent, in a collective formation, in a subcultural scene, I had to find out who I was as an artist individually. I also needed a job. Matthew Higgs, who I had known in London, was working at the Wattis Institute at that time and co-chairing the MFA at California College of the Arts with Lydia Matthews. In 2004 he introduced me to Lydia, and I was suddenly teaching again and meeting artists based here. I am still grateful—Matthew is one of those people who continues to open doors for others.

Reading speculative fiction was great preparation for a triplet pregnancy and for life with three infants. While pregnant I entertained the thought that I might not need to make art anymore once they were born, but it quickly became very obvious that it was the other way around. I felt that they would never know me if I didn't do my work and that without it I would be a terrible and frustrated mother. I gave up residual ambivalence about calling myself an artist, and even about the artworld itself. I had worked in a bunch of different spheres by then, which made it easier to see that the big systemic social problems occur in every field. It began to make sense that I grappled with them in the field at the center of my desire—by doing what mattered to me most. I recall this moment of clarity so vividly because it has had such a great impact. When I have doubts now, I take it as a message from the universe, asking me to confront something or make a change.

Being in a position where I had to fight to make time for my work meant I no longer took being an artist for granted. Many days I felt I was trying to do the impossible—to be a working artist as a mother of triplets, a now older woman of color, without a corporate income. I took a semester and summer off from teaching when I gave birth in 2006, but all I could do was video myself reading the babies theory and science fiction while breast-feeding. I thought a lot about sustenance and ecosystems. I began to work with imagery from Indian mythology, recognizing how Eurocentric my art education had been, and to build visual languages to embody cultural hybridity and creolization. Then, and to this day, I draw on the wisdom of my holistic doctor Gabrielle Francis, who I began working with seventeen years ago. She exemplifies the potential of combining knowledge systems, self-care, and doing things your own way, on your own time.

I also had financial support that I never had previously. My partner was able to buy an apartment and I was in a position to teach part time and still pay for some child-care. Were it not for that I am sure we could not have stayed in San Francisco with three kids. Mike has a physical disability, which added a layer of complexity, but he was doing a lot of the cooking and laundry while I worked outside of the house. His support afforded me some time to develop the language and ideas of my work even with kids and teaching. This relatively stable situation also allowed me to feel, and deeply appreciate, the generative energy of children, despite the hard work and physical exhaustion. Through them I feel an expanded connection to the world, to time, and to the questions posed by the future. Motherhood is a portal and a form of futurism.

Between 2003, when I returned to the United States, and 2008, when my kids went to preschool, I went back to the basic questions—what do I want and need to make and what kind of artist am I? I worked in obscurity for several years. When I began to find a visual language things started to happen with my career. In 2008 I began to feel that it was time for a studio outside the house. I applied for and got a fellowship at Kala Art Institute, which culminated in a 2009 exhibition. Betti-Sue

Hertz was, at that time, director of visual arts at the Yerba Buena Center for the Arts (YBCA) in San Francisco. She saw my Kala exhibition and sent Julio César Morales, who was an adjunct curator at YBCA, for a studio visit. They were considering artists for *Bay Area Now 6*, their triennial survey exhibition, and ended up including my work. Julio is an amazing artist whose work I admire greatly; he is also a curator whose support has been instrumental for me as for so many other artists. He recommended my work to the gallerist Wendi Norris whom he had recently started working with. She came to do a studio visit and offered to represent me despite the fact that I had no commercial visibility then. Gallery Wendi Norris has recently published the first monograph of my work, covering nine years of my painting, hybrid film, and installation work. The book began in 2011 with my first museum project commissioned by the San Jose Museum of Art. My collaborative history has followed me in my studio projects, with the understanding that no art becomes public without collective production. I learn from all the people I work with, both at the gallery and from curators such as Jodi Throckmorton, Marc Mayer, and Claudia Schmuckli, with whom I have done major projects. Recently, choreographer Hope Mohr and I are bringing together dancers and immigrant and refugee artists to work across disciplines, using speculative fiction as a process to imagine new futures, in performance and film.

The current iteration of my life is full of abundance and challenge. I have many more opportunities as an artist to be part of a larger conversation. I enjoy a full-time studio practice and a steady flow of exhibitions, commissioned projects, residencies, and speaking engagements. Over time I have gained confidence in my process, even in the (necessary) time spent being lost. This past fall (2023) after a pandemic-related postponement, I was able to open *Time Warriors,* my first exhibition of paintings in New York, hosted by Wendi Norris, which brought my new work into conversation with works by the surrealist artist Alice Rahon. Having this visual dialogue was profound in many ways, notable for the context of this essay is that she was less than 30 years older than me when she passed. I am at a pivotal moment, my kids nearing high school graduation and considering what my next chapter will look like.

I was recently awarded tenure at the California College of the Arts, where I serve as chair of the film programs and teach in the graduate fine art program. Essentially, I have two full careers and three teenagers. It feels like I have been doing the same thing for a long time, except everything I care about has scaled up and expanded in many directions or taken a different shape. For most of my teaching career I worked a part-time schedule, which meant I could just about juggle everything with young kids. I have always seen my students as artists who are simply at an earlier point in their development. I love looking at their work and talking to artists about how they think about what they are doing. After graduation, students quickly become fellow artists.

Now my kids are much more independent, but I have also become the single earner supporting my children due to Mike's health issues. My overhead is very high, particularly with the unconscionable cost of living in San Francisco, so I need both studio and teaching income to make ends meet. Professional growth in both realms has come at the right time. Tenure affords me better pay and sabbatical privileges in addition to summers for much-needed breaks. Chairing is a different kind of commitment, which sometimes has the benefits of more remote work and autonomy of my schedule. I enjoy being able to create programming, bring in artists and filmmakers, and recommending new adjunct professors. However, higher education has changed a lot in my time as a faculty member and the administrative demands can be a distraction from an artistic mission. It requires a specific kind of vigilance, both to keep artistic work at the center of focus of our programs and to have good boundaries that protect my health and my time (which are really the same thing). In 2023, I was able, for the first time, to hire a more regular studio assistant and to earn slightly more as an artist than I did in my professorship. It feels like a turning of the tide.

I have so many questions that drive my artwork and my sense of the future. I feel like I am in the midst of another major shift with my children nearing college age. Having two full-time careers is not entirely sustainable or satisfying long term without the correct support. I frequently call in my intention to maintain presence; to resist being coerced into exhaustion. I made myself a promise a long time ago that I would continue to protect my ability to feel the energetic and multidimensional experiences of time that fuel a creative life—even when culture pushes against it or extremely difficult and upsetting things are going down. I am committed to making artwork in order to live fully, stay open to the unexpected, connect to sense and sensation, reconfigure relationships, and picture differently tuned worlds. •

# ROMY ACHITUV

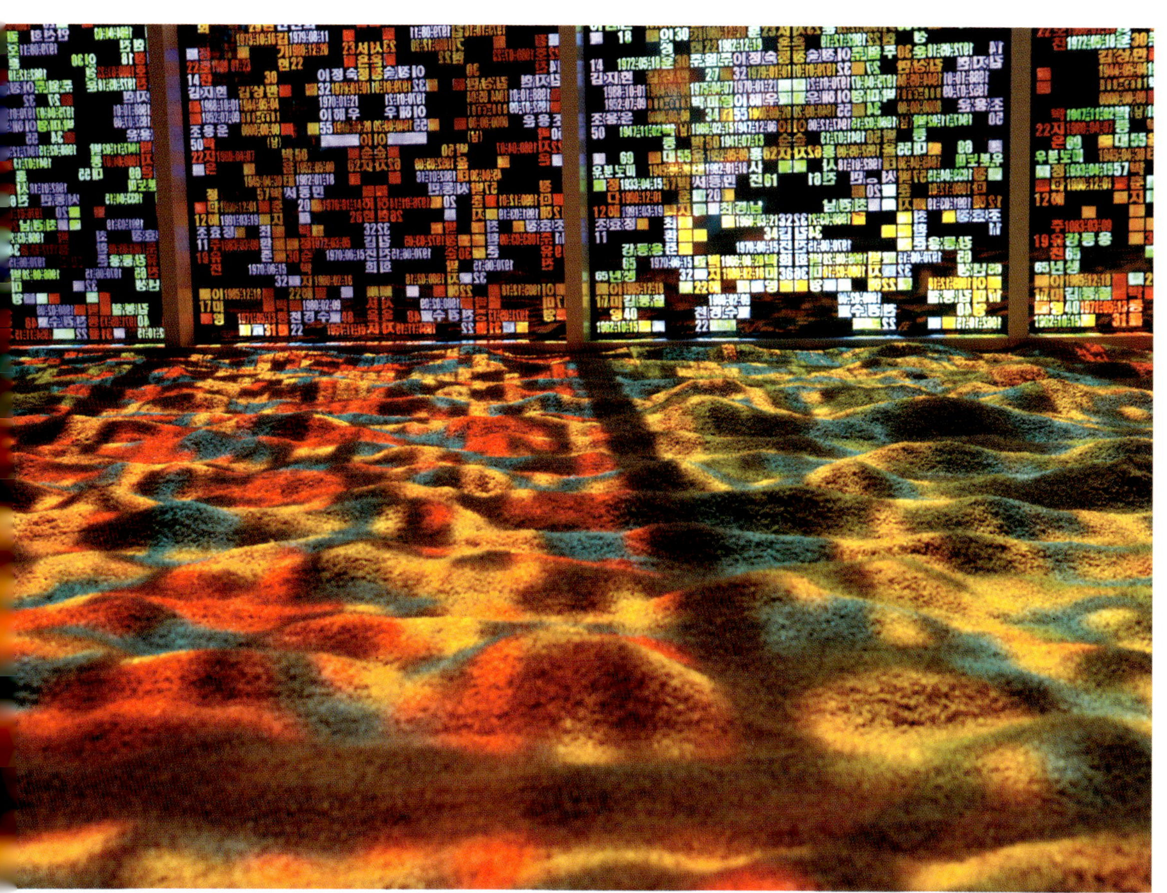

MY ENGAGEMENT with art was, in many ways, an inheritance from the labyrinthine tapestry of my family's emotional history. My earliest memories are of a home filled with art and opera, and a sense of reality merging with the surreal, reflecting the ways my parents related to their turbulent pasts.

My father, a young Polish student who emigrated to Palestine, served in the British Army during World War II, a time marked by the loss of his entire family in the Holocaust. In a twist of fate, he married a young woman he had recruited to teach in one of the Jewish schools he founded in Italy at the end of the war. Their union bore a tragic secret: a crippled child from a failed abortion attempt, which may or may not have been known to my father. This child, my half-brother, was cared for in a convent home near Trieste, Northern Italy. Despite their divorce, my father, together with the child's grandparents, shared the responsibility of caring for the boy until his untimely death in his early twenties. I learned of his existence by accident one day in my twenties, poking through old documents in boxes in our apartment's storage space. I never found a way to broach the topic with my father.

What I knew of my mother's life was equally complex, rooted in her idiosyncratic upbringing in an unorthodox-yet-orthodox Jewish home. Her father, my grandfather, was deeply religious yet liberal-minded, and encouraged her artistic talents, allowing her to sing on the budding national radio in the 1930s, an act

Romy Achituv
*Memory Stain,* a memorial installation for the victims of the Daegu 2003 subway fire
2014
6x6x6m
Mixed-media (vinyl stickers, stained glass paint on acetate, rice husk)
Courtesy of the artist

considered sacrilegious by religious standards. He was also a fervent political and social activist, advocating and fundraising for the large orphanage he administered in Jerusalem. He returned from his international travels with art books filled with European masterpieces, works deemed heretical by his community for their nudity and Christian iconography. My mother brought her artistic passions to her first marriage to a young poet, a Holocaust survivor whose life ended abruptly when he died of a brain tumor in his early thirties. My sister and I grew up in the shadow of this man, idolized by my mother, a figure of lost potential and profound grief.

Our family home was a blend of these cultures and hidden traumas. My mother's manic exuberance contrasted starkly with my father's gentle melancholy. We navigated an emotional landscape marked by loss and pain, some known explicitly, some merely intuited. Despite, or perhaps because of, the secrets and unknown crannies of our family's history, there was an underlying current of support for my artistic endeavors. Perhaps it was the recognition of art's power to make sense of the insensible that led my parents to encourage my pursuit of this passion.

The long shadows cast by my parents' past were periodically dispelled by my mother's formidable life force. Her profusions of creative works ranged from her transgressive early singing career to a late-in-life discovery of her talent as a stained glass artist and stone carver. My parents' idiosyncrasies, their unspoken histories, my mother's perpetually embellished and reinvented universe, my father's poorly masked fragility, were the colors with which I painted my world. It was in this environment, rich in enigmas, that I developed an attachment to the fabricated image as holding the promise of grounding my narratives and understanding of reality. Art was a source of life in my childhood household, but encountering the way it was taught and discussed outside of my family was a startling experience.

My initial encounter with the artworld was in the tiny microcosm of my art academy as a young sculpture student at the Bezalel Academy of Arts and Design in Jerusalem. As an innocent first-year student, new to the machinations of this unique subculture, I was lost navigating the cliques that divided our small fine arts department. Confused by ideological battles waged over my head while ostensibly making claims about my and my peers' work, I receded into my studio, clinging to some unidentified intuition to guide me through the discursive fog I was stumbling around in.

In some ways, this alienating environment was itself the best art schooling I could have asked for, inadvertently reinforcing a drive toward self-reliance. This initially manifested in a contrarian instinct that directed my creative focus toward making choices that my passions endowed with conviction. Going with what "just felt right," I pursued figurative and representational work in an art department where this type of practice was borderline taboo. Still driven to make figurative work all these decades later, I understand the choice to adhere to my primary artistic direction as having been fundamentally self-preserving.

After graduating in 1985, I pursued academic studies in philosophy at the Hebrew University in Jerusalem in an attempt to acquire tools I hoped would allow me to make some sense of the conceptual mayhem I had been immersed in. At the same time, I felt encouraged by a small burst of public recognition in the form of a studio residency, a couple prizes, and invitations to participate in group shows. Given that I could cover my expenses working part time as a security guard, I was fairly confident that I could find a way to sustain an artistic practice.

As friends began settling down and starting families, I remained focused on making art. In 1989, I moved to New York to attend a graduate program in figurative sculpture at the New York Academy of Art, and survival no longer seemed assured. The cost of living was astronomical compared to Jerusalem, and by 1993 I had already left a couple ill-suited art schools without completing a degree and was continuously scavenging for odd jobs: painting houses, moving, gardening, secretarial work. I may have been content with that lifestyle had I been able to consistently produce, but I was so depleted by the demands of daily existence that for a long while my highest creative achievement was the stealth sleeping rigs I constructed in my Alphabet City studio: a table that doubled as a bed and closet, and workstations that provided additional clandestine storage space. During the mid-1990s, the years that New Yorkers now see as a great era of bygone real estate possibilities, I was illegally squatting in that office-space-turned-artist-studio/darkroom, which reeked of developer solution and gasoline from the trucking garage downstairs, and scraping by working for minimum wage as a switchboard operator and as an utterly unqualified counselor for mentally ill homeless teens and adults. Trapped by my circumstances, I was treading water with no foreseeable escape.

Though I had neither energy nor time for studio work, I continued, as I had for years, to carry my Nikon FM2 with me wherever I went and to randomly document my surroundings. Around this time, I also began tinkering with a video camera a friend had purchased for her own projects, and I grew intrigued by its digital effects features, which I very roughly began to also explore in my photographs. My friend was attending Interactive Telecommunications Program (ITP), NYU's ever-evolving graduate media-communication program, which was focused at the time on new media technologies, and my fresh yet very rudimentary familiarity with digital tools ignited a sense of new possibilities. In 1995 I enrolled in the program, envisioning it as essentially a vocational school that would provide me with the skills to fashion an escape route from the life I was living.

While I initially imagined that I would emerge from the program with a profession and a livelihood, I soon realized that I was neither sufficiently efficient to be a professional designer, nor sufficiently gifted to compete as a technologist in the commercial design or programming world. The introduction to digital technologies, however, fueled my imagination. It became evident to me that in order to sustain my commitment and focus in the program I would have to treat it as an art school, and the digital tools I was playing with as an extension of my creative palette. From this perspective, every small exercise became a playful creative challenge.

My return to school also reintroduced me to that great American institution of federally funded indentured servitude, i.e., student loans. I no longer had a long-term financial strategy nor faith that I would ever have the means to pay back my accumulating debt, but I nonetheless embraced the opportunity of a temporary respite from survival woes, proceeding down this yellow brick road toward an uncertain future. My sole concern was the time and project financing I was acquiring.

This *modus operandi* could have landed me in a precarious place, but as I was wrapping up my studies, a friend and classmate I had collaborated with, Camille Utterback, tenaciously pursued opportunities to exhibit our interactive installation, *Text Rain*. We surprisingly and unwittingly found ourselves sought after by new media festivals, museums, and collectors, both domestically and internationally.

The initial broad interest in this one particular artwork led to a series of invitations to exhibit additional works, and to proliferating opportunities. Following suit were international teaching positions and public commissions that soon allowed me to pay off the six-figure debt I had blithely amassed. What I had imagined was going to be the fashioning of a practical skillset ended up blossoming into an actual creative practice.

My creative digital-media work continued to evolve, slowly expanding toward interdisciplinary projects and commissions, leading to the co-founding in 1998 of ARTEAM, a small arts collective in Israel, and to initiatives that took on a much more active element of social and political engagement. The communal aspect of my work became meaningful and grounding in a way I had not expected. While affording a source for material sustenance it also provided an emotional anchor outside of myself, lifting me beyond the narrow confines of my struggles as an independent artist.

Still, while the trajectory of my practice generated income opportunities, income opportunities directed my practice trajectory. I was caught up in a cycle, which while rich in its diversity, was constricted by the boundaries of my previous work and public image. It was easier to find a teaching position in digital media-technology than in fine art, easier to apply for funding for a project with a media component than to finance personal work that had no clear grounding in my new media portfolio.

Throughout all those years, however, I longed to return to sculpture and to a creative process that was more intimate and unmediated. I gradually began introducing tactile materials into my projects, which also grew increasingly sculptural. Finally, after more than two and a half decades split between three continents, I managed to take the savings I earned during those years and in 2016 I rented a sculpture studio at the Old American Can Factory in Brooklyn.

In the years that followed, life began feeling different in some fundamental ways. I penned the first draft of this essay around that time. I had recently gotten married and became a father, and could finally afford to pay rent for a place to sleep outside of my studio. Looking back, I see the way the emotional and financial grounding I attained enabled not just my return to sculpture but also my pursuit of a stable and meaningful personal life. At the same time, on a day-to-day basis, it was a solitary pursuit, and as I labored in my studio, feeling my way through that old familiar medium, I found myself re-experiencing insecurities I had as a younger artist, and seeing more clearly the struggles that defined me then.

As it happened, that period of life was upended during the COVID-19 pandemic. We left Brooklyn for California and then Boston as my wife pursued training opportunities for her doctorate in clinical psychology. I packed my studio into boxes and I am still figuring out how to return. Our one child led to another, and while these gorgeous, funny sprites have brought a never-dreamed-of dimension of joy and beauty to my life, the financial reality of pursuing a sculpture practice is just as daunting now as it was in New York in the 1990s.

One of the takeaways from my years of wandering between mediums is learning that I can work (and think and "speak") in a variety of media. While my wife's career lends a measure of financial stability to our family, my own artistic survival requires me to be nimble in my pursuit of creative outlets. These days I am primarily seeking opportunities in the public realm and as a teacher. I long to return to the solace of my studio work, but with two small boys in tow, the stakes of pursuing an artistic life have never been higher.

# SONIA BAEZ-HERNANDEZ

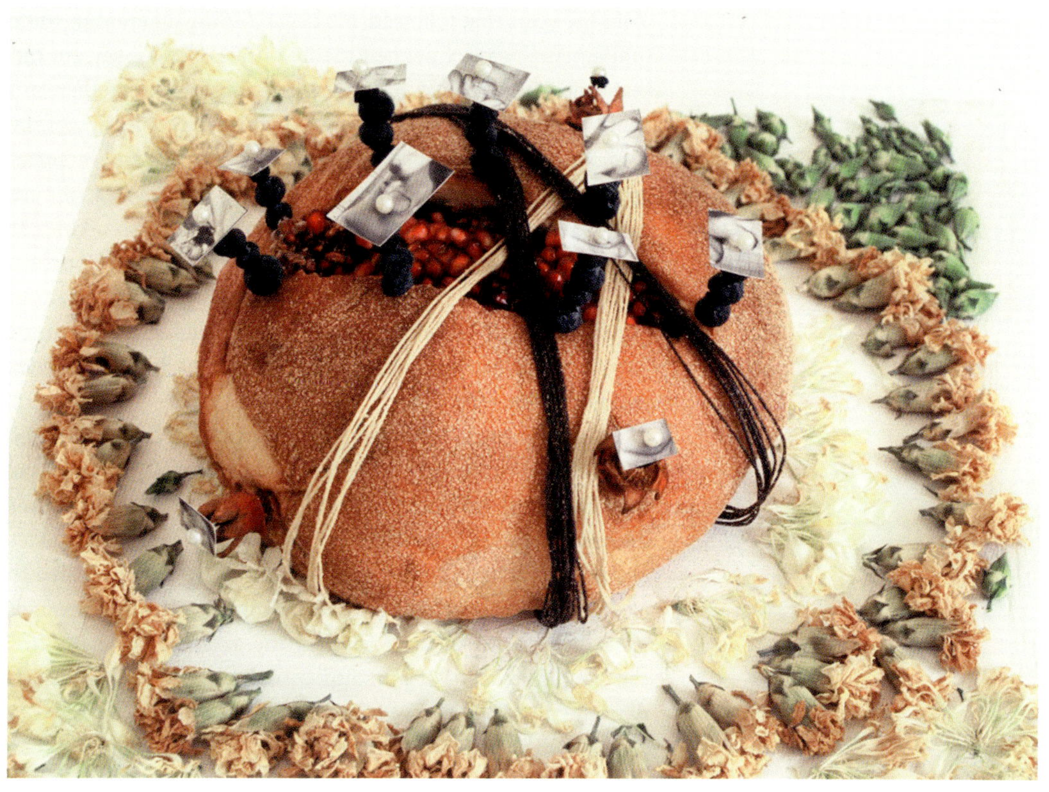

TO SUSTAIN MY artistic career, I am dependent on full-time employment. I was among many teachers who lost their jobs in Florida in 2022. The neo-inquisition of the Florida state government began by banning library books, restricting curriculums, and eradicating academic freedom, research, and critical thinking. Parents in the state criticized artistic projects inspired by social practice and art research; it became difficult to participate in art competitions. School administrators advanced anti-diversity and limitations of academic freedom with a mandate.

The State of Florida's exclusion of diversity takes the form of re-appropriating colonialism and race/ethnicity, censorship of feminism, and LGBTQ oppressions that re-constitute dangerous groups, inequalities, stigmas, and the subjugation of diverse groups.

From 2019 to 2020, Florida's Department of Economic Education Opportunity (DEO) used technology, broken by design, to make it impossible for me to file an unemployment claim. After I experienced weeks of receiving errors from the authentication portal (like in the film *Metropolis* and *Brazil*), I quit, saving myself more humiliation by continuing to go through such an arduous process.

In August 2020, the landlord increased my rent. Because he overcharged me for years, I opposed the increase. I knew this as the real estate in my neighborhood was cheaper. I had to pay the

Sonia Beaz-Hernandez
*Reconstruction I*
2001
4″x15″x4.2″
Fibers decaying, ten scars
contact/prints
Courtesy of the artist
Photography by Diana Solis

rent that he demanded. In 2023, Miami's inflation ranking was the highest in the United States.

I was working in a factory part-time when I was offered a teaching position that required me to work twice a week, four hours each day, to supplement my income. Because the hours of teaching conflicted with my hours working at the factory, I asked my manager for a change in hours working at the factory. He rejected my request. So I left the job at the factory and accepted the teaching position for $50 an hour.

Even though I have some employment and a place to live, I felt deprived as I lost my studio and access to art materials. This affected my artistic practice. Like the siblings in *The House Taken Over* by Julio Cortázar, I felt anxiety, fear, and isolation.

For some relief, my friend Aida Tejada allowed me to use her studio while she was taking classes in the morning. Working in Aida's studio gave me hope for stability while navigating my feeling of emptiness and letting go. For three months I painted and documented the paintings to apply for a grant to have a studio and receive materials. I was also busy working on my website and applying for jobs in Chicago. Being unsettled in my personal life affected my professional life. For example, I got an invitation to participate in a group exhibition. Because I could not access my storage space, it made it impossible for me to participate.

*****

My mom, Francisca Hernandez, applied for her green card in the 1960s, seeking a future for herself and her five children. We immigrated from the Dominican Republic to Puerto Rico to realize new opportunities and dreams. She was a single mother.

I am a woman of African heritage. When I was a child studying in a Puerto Rican school, they assigned me and my younger brother to the same grade. I had challenges with reading and writing, so I referred to mnemonics and different learning styles to help me along. I played guitar, sang in the chorus, wrote poetry, and graduated with honors.

Teachers targeted my race, accent, the way I dressed, and my coiled hair. One day in class, the teacher demonstrated her disdain for me when she pinch-gripped my skin and said, "Go back to the Dominican Republic." She pinched me several times in the classroom. That experience shattered me. I still remember the time I left school crying. I walked a mile or so, noticed the unfamiliar landscape, and felt lost. I eventually retraced my way back to school. Over time, my accent became acculturated.

In 1984, I earned a BA from the University of Puerto Rico (UPR). While at UPR, I took a drawing class and an art history course. I remember access to modern art and contemporary artists' works were limited to books and magazines. I was also the president of the Political Science Association, implementing a series of conferences on culture, politics, and literature.

I met Rubén Rivera Matos while commuting from Río Piedras to Bayamón on Pisa y Corre. He was an artist and philosophy student at UPR. We had a friendship and frequent dialogue about abstraction, figuration, philosophy, music, and politics. I have fond memories of our experiences together including joining protesters objecting to tuition increases at UPR and assisting Rubén with painting a mural, which evoked images of Picasso's *Guernica*. I took my first drawing class with Professor Luisa Géigel Brunet. We were fascinated by her teaching, sharing her drawings, and her narrations of the architectural transformation of the old San Juan.

*****

From 1984 to 1990, I lived in New York City and experimented with drawing, collage, and mixed media. In 1990, I enrolled in graduate classes at the University of California Los Angeles. In 1992, I received an MA in Sociology from UCLA. My thesis was titled "The Constitution of Graffiti as a Crime."

From 1992–93, I was honored with a Critical Studies Fellowship to attend the Paris Program in Critical Theory as a researcher at the Michel Foucault Center. I listened to Foucault's lectures from the archive, read unpublished lectures, documents, and books, and accessed other works on subjectivity and governmentality, self-care, literature analysis, and philosophy. Of the articles I wrote and presented from my time in Paris, I wrote an article on graffiti, tracing the practice of appropriation from popular culture, and an article on self-care in the Phaedrus philosophy influenced by Foucault, Pierre Hadot, and others. At the same time, I experimented with stone lithography in Paris with my friends Fernando Puig Rosado and Nancy, and created a series of drawings and wrote poems.

In 1995, my nephew Alex called me and asked if he could live with me in Los Angeles. At the time, I was an associate researcher at UCLA, researching the impact of education in Black and Brown communities in the inner city. Alex lived with me from 1994–95 and attended school in Los Angeles. In 1996, we moved to Chicago so I could earn my MFA at the School of the Art Institute of Chicago (SAIC).

During my first year at SAIC, I taught sociology and was a research assistant while attending school. Alex was 13. He would meet me at SAIC and attend art critiques, commenting about the works that the class critiqued. I remember one day he said, "I am more popular than you at SAIC." I looked at him, and we smiled.

In my second year, I worked full time as a training manager at the National Coalition for Latinxs with Disabilities. After graduating from SAIC in 1998, I met with a group of women in my apartment in Chicago. We formed a collective named the Rooted Nomad. We wrote, read, and performed together. We hosted poetry workshops for students at the Children's Museum in Chicago and other venues, received limited compensation, and divided it among ourselves. In 1999, Karen Sorensen and I submitted a proposal to perform for a juried group show called *Connections* at SAIC's Gallery 2. We developed choreography, concept, stone percussion, and vocal sounds and performed *The Tear Holder*. I started to work with the University of Illinois Chicago and on community projects with the Museum of Contemporary Art Chicago from 1999 to 2001. I developed a curriculum to introduce contemporary art to third- and sixth-grade students. The students' projects represented their Latino identity and culture.

*****

In April 2001, I was diagnosed with breast cancer. While facing breast cancer, I recalled the powerful, political photography of Jo Spence, who had documented her personal battle with breast cancer. I was one of 45 million uninsured Americans, impacted by the violation of human rights. I collected documentation revealing my body modifications and other documents supporting these violations. This activism inspired me to embrace the collective impact of health disparities. My projects interrogating the culture of illness, gender crisis, and medical gaze came together in a documentary about dehumanization from my experience.

My friends Laura and Markeza sought a second opinion for me. Frances Aparicio edited my complaint for the violation of patient rights. My family traveled to support me before and after surgery. Lisa Brock called our mutual friend Peter Sporn, a professor of medicine, to help me obtain good care. He took the time to select a team of medical professionals: Seema Khan, William Gardishar, and Julius Few. They responded to my medical needs, cared for me as a human being, and answered my questions, which helped facilitate my research and contributed to my art installations about breast cancer.

Days before my biopsy, I packed up the apartment to move back to Florida. At night I read with tears between my hands. As a result of the biopsy, the only choice was a mastectomy. I appreciated the support of my friends and family during the recovery. As my mom left to board her flight at the airport, we said our goodbyes and fought back our tears.

In sadness, I moved to Esther Soler and Marc Zimmerman's apartment. They became part of my family. During my recovery, Esther provided me with comfort and rest, which enabled me to take the loop for appointments. My friend Lisa was my chemo companion.

In 2001, before I moved to Florida, Marc edited my application for the Pollock-Krasner Foundation grant. In Florida, it was impossible to have medical insurance if you had pre-existing conditions. Therefore, I had to travel to Chicago from Florida for five years to receive treatment for breast cancer.

I was honored with a Pollock-Krasner Foundation grant in 2002 and it sustained my life and artistic career. The award allowed me to have a creative practice without interruption for a year. I produced twenty drawings, 25 installations, twenty paintings, and two fiber pieces that year in a rented studio. In 2003, I had the opportunity to curate *Body as a Poetic Space* in Chicago.

My medical appointments inspired the opportunity to organize two panels on breast cancer and prevention, sponsored by the University of Illinois Chicago's Lectures in Communities series, thanks to Frances Aparicio, who organized the discussions and helped me secure funding.

Lisa introduced me to Jean Rene, an SAIC alumnus and a filmmaker who agreed to work with me on an independent film project, *Territories of the Breast*. This film featured women in conversation about breast cancer, the experiences of breast cancer, the uninsured, gender, resistance to inequality, and access to health care. The first version of *Territories of the Breast* was 158 minutes and released in 2006.

My first screening of the documentary was at Columbia College in Chicago. At the time, there was a dispute over who was the director of the film. Rene argued this as I tried to negotiate with him. He edited and videographed the film but did not direct *Territories of the Breast*. I was the creator and director of this film. Rene showed his disappointment by acting unethically and the pandemic didn't help, either. I saw that he was selling my documentary on Amazon without giving me any profits, claimed a prize designated for me, took credit for the film when he had no right to and he was interviewed about the documentary with a friend who had no role in contributing to the film.

Unfortunately, even though I copyrighted *Territories of the Breast*, I did not have a written agreement with Rene on his role in the development of the film. This was a lesson for me. Trusting this person was not enough. However, it was only fair to share profits with each person who contributed in making the film. This was my promise. I also advocated for Jean Rene and paid for his transportation to film interviews, purchased tapes, equipment, etc., but still he acted unethically. I also learned that I needed a budget for materials, a salary for myself and assistants as well as money for lodging and transportation, among many other expenses. This is now my practice after this experience.

I started caring for my mom in 2012 because she was afraid to be alone. After receiving a second opinion, it was confirmed that my mother had Alzheimer's disease. My brother Andre was in denial. I was her primary caregiver for a year, arriving at 6:30 a.m. every day, assisting her with shopping, doctor's appointments, and everything else meeting her needs.

While caring for my mother, I taught four courses as an adjunct faculty member at Broward College. I kept applying for opportunities including an artist-in-residence program with the Service Employees International Union (SEIU) to create artwork in collaboration with the workers for a convention. My mom was living with Andre. I would take her to radiation treatments, senior Zumba and yoga classes.

I called the manager to request a payment extension for September's rent. She responded, "Pay the rent by September 15th, or you will receive eviction papers." I complained to the Affordable Housing for Artists organization, but they could not help.

In 2013, I sold my car to get by. I used my brother's car to take my mom to her treatments and continue as her caregiver despite my situation. At the same time, I installed my solo exhibition *Embodiment and the Medical Gaze* at the University of Miami Gallery.

*****

At an artist residency in Kalamazoo, Michigan, I started drawing and researching for work inspired by human rights, health disparities, and healing for a new series of installations. I also developed a performance concept, costume design, installations and a poem titled "The Flesh." Curated with Teresa Vasquez, the performance captured her unique cadence and her music.

In 2014, Curator Morgana Wallace Cooper invited me to curate an exhibition in Ajo, Arizona, with the International Sonoran Desert Alliance (ISDA). I worked remotely and sent documentation while we discussed and envisioned ideas for the exhibition *Redrawing Borders — Art Activist, Humanitarian, and Ecological.* We worked effectively while I was caring for my mom.

*****

For artists to receive opportunities, (such as artist-in-residence programs, teaching, curatorial projects, and more) involves engagement with networks of different organizations, professors, activists, curators, and others who generate revenue. I have received opportunities through recommendations by cultural organizers who know my work. Sometimes these connections alleviate joblessness and financial anxiety. However, they are temporary and not the answer to the overall displacement that I continue to experience.

When finding housing and basic necessities during precarious times, the option is to move to a post-studio situation and a different, varied contemporary art practice. My interdisciplinary practice allows me to work with other mediums, such as fiber and found objects. I can make sculptures, assemblage, perform and create installations. While my art supplies and archived works were in boxes, I felt nostalgia for specific works and discourse.

In addition to not having a stable life, I am concerned about aging. I hope my skills, experience, and training will be valued. Individuals can experience discrimination in any of these social categories: aging, race, ethnicity, gender, a foreign accent, and disabilities. Unfortunately, institutions discriminate based on their values. Aging, in my case, could cause more micro-aggressions, stereotypes, and exclusion.

Regarding teaching throughout my life, my experience as an adjunct professor has been financially thwarted. As an adjunct, I was always paid below the poverty line, and yet I did so much more than what I was asked to do because the students deserved more than what I was paid to do. This is the norm in higher education: institutions are paying people unfairly and create a hierarchy that is not inclusive.

I am continually deprived of housing and security due to marginalization. Being deprived of these fundamental rights and access to necessities that are essential for living, it is challenging for me to create work for exhibitions and perform worldwide. It's important to recognize sustainability is unequal and there should be access for those who are unrepresented in all aspects. •

# SONYA KELLIHER-COMBS

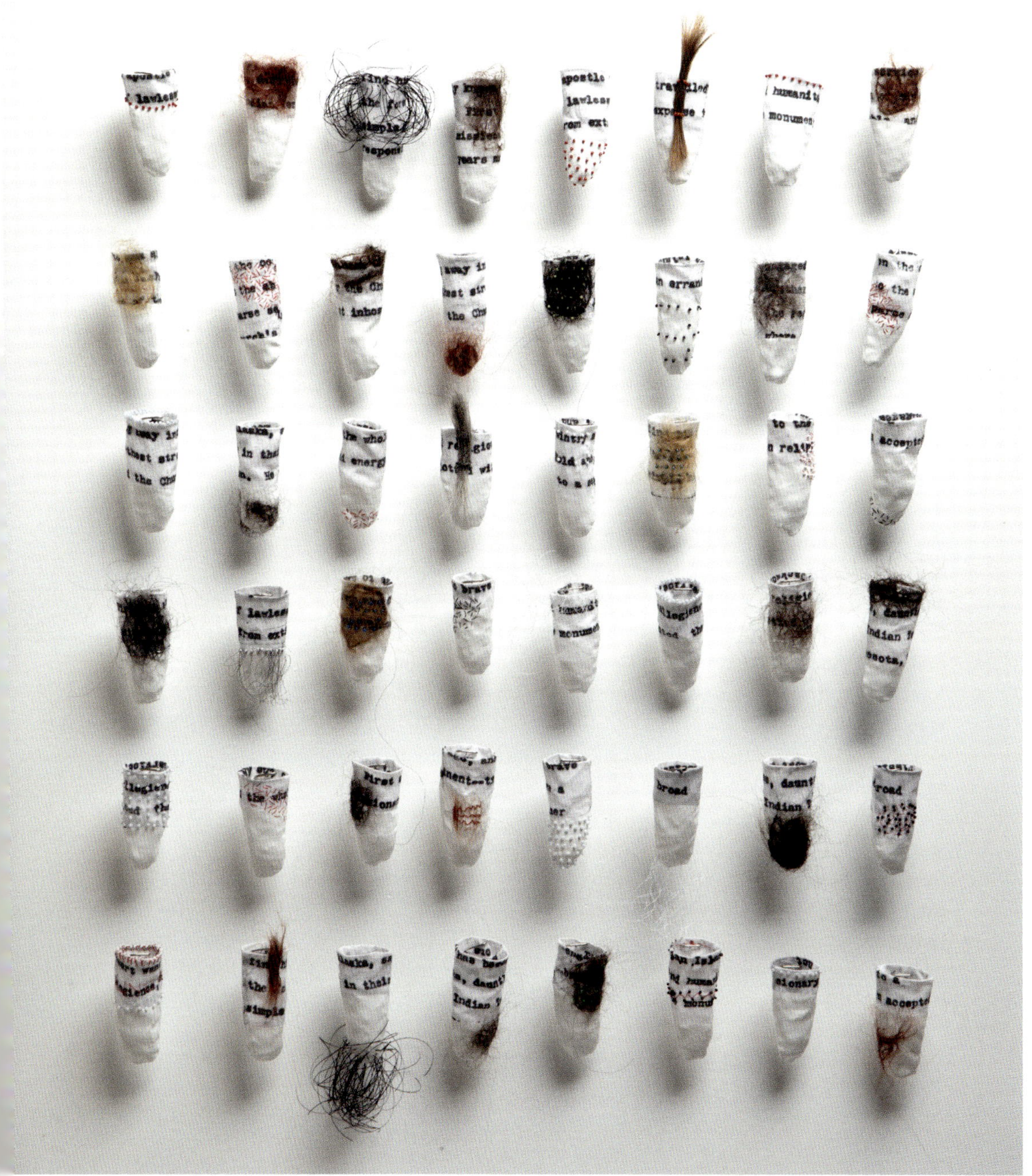

GROWING UP in Nome, Alaska, I spent summers at our camp where we worked, hunted, and gathered food and supplies for the winter. It was there where I learned to listen; listened to learn from family, community members, and nature. I am of mixed descent: Athabascan, Iñupiaq, Irish, German, Scottish, and Danish. My cultural background and identity are at the forefront of my work and life. Through observation and the practice of time-honored traditions—skin sewing, beading, and food preparation—I realized my role as woman, daughter, sister, wife and artist.

I am the second oldest of six kids, and very lucky to be a part of a big close family. We are a blended family with four children from my mom Trudy Kelliher's first marriage, two from her second and three from my fathers' marriages. I am fortunate to have both a dad, Patrick Kelliher, who raised us, and a father, Jim Stotts. Today it is more commonplace, but as kids we were one of the few divorced families. I am thankful every day for my mom's strength and love and for the great gift of having both a dad and father.

I grew up without the concept of art, art as a job or career. In our home art was infused into our life. My mom has always been a creative person, making our clothes, outdoor gear, foods, etc. Growing up, money was scarce, so many things were handmade. In many Indigenous cultures there was no word for art. It makes

Sonya Kelliher-Combs
*Small Secrets, Sheldon Jackson*
2021
Dimensions variable
Printed fabric, glass beed, human hair, steel pen, nylon thread
Courtesy of the artist
Photography by Chris Arend

sense when you study our historical objects: objects imbued with spirit, adornment meant to empower them.

When I was a young girl, I was afraid to go to my first day of school. My father gave me a beautiful object, an ancient harpoon toggle. He told me it would make me strong and help me get over my fear of the first day. I still remember crying, but I can't imagine how hard it would have been had I not had my talisman. Still today when I need to be brave I wear it. Something courses through that small implement that helps ground and connect me to something bigger than me.

Throughout my childhood, I was drawn to creating; I loved putting things together, making in the 1970s and 1980s. One teacher in particular had a huge influence on me at Nome-Beltz High School, Dottie Sanders. She was a transplant from New Jersey and New York, full of adventure and spirit. Mrs. Sanders was always nurturing but also challenging. She encouraged us to think outside of the box. Her adventurous spirit was contagious. Although she has since passed, I still hear her voice inside my head urging me forward—to not be afraid to speak the truth.

Other large influences during grade school and high school were two generous elders, Edna Alvanna and Harry Koozata, who worked within our schools sharing art and culture. Anna Gologergan was an amazing culture bearer who taught me the endangered art of processing marine mammal gut during my college years; this is my favorite medium to work with. I can still remember her small smile when my younger sister and I brought her our first butchered walrus stomach. She asked, "What did you do?" She quickly hung the stomach from a hook placed in the middle of her kitchen, and the weight of the stomach hung to the floor. She quietly made quick work of de-fleshing the outside of the stomach and handed over the knife for us to complete the task. She invited me to come over whenever I wanted, and she would share. I am forever thankful for these generous lessons.

We grew up in a Catholic household. My mother, Trudy Hildebrand Kelliher, is from the interior Athabascan village of Nulato, a small town situated on the banks of the Yukon River. It is one of many Alaska Native villages that was claimed by the Catholic church during the early Western settling of Alaska.

My dad, Patrick Kelliher, is first generation from Ireland. Years growing up Catholic have included both good and bad experiences in our family. Several series of my work comment on the entangled struggles of Alaska Natives and the church, including those addressing abuse and suicide. Alaska Natives are three times more likely to take their own life than the rest of our nation. In a new survey taken by the Department of Justice, 84% of Native American and Alaska Native women have experienced violence, and 56% have experienced sexual violence. I believe we need to voice these issues in order to transform them and promote healing. It is something that I endeavor to address in my work.

Although I had a rich creative upbringing, I never thought I would become an artist. I was going to be a lawyer or maybe an engineer. In 1987, I graduated high school as valedictorian with a full scholarship to the University of Alaska Fairbanks where I started my college experience. It was there that I took my first drawing class with instructor David Mollet. It was a hard class, probably one of the most difficult I have ever taken. The first day, he was not encouraging. Rambling on about the life of an artist he flatly stated, "Only one of you will be making art in twenty years." I can't explain it but somehow knew it would be me. I changed my major and received my bachelor of fine arts in 1992.

After my undergraduate studies, I spent 100 days traveling around Europe with a good friend. It was transformative experiencing all the history, art, and culture I had studied and viewed only by projector slides for so many years. When I came home, I was ripe to create. The next three years I worked a full-time job and painted. In that time period I had two solo exhibitions and was invited to participate in the first important exhibition of my career, *Arts from the Arctic*. This exhibition was a multinational, traveling exhibition representing the diverse Indigenous arts from the Arctic and was curated by Indigenous artists and scholars from the circumpolar North, including the Iñupiaq artist Ronald Senungetuk. Ron, considered the father of contemporary Alaska Native art, became a friend and mentor.

My high school sweetheart and future husband, Shaun Combs, and I moved back to Nome in 1994, and I worked as a tutor at our local grade school. It was great to be back home with my family, community, and the land that I love, but it was also difficult to be away from my college arts community and to find time to focus on painting. It was one of the most trying periods in my art life: it was difficult to get supplies, shipping was more than the cost of my paint, and the dialogue I had grown accustomed to was non-existent. I taught a class at the Northwest Community College, and it pushed me to apply to graduate school.

Looking for diversity and close proximity to home in a graduate school, I applied to schools on the West Coast. I chose to pursue my MFA at Arizona State University. Throughout the program I was met with both support and opposition. A fellow graduate student told me the only reason I was there was because I was a minority. Growing up I had experienced racism being called "dirty little Indian" or "Muktuk eater"— I was not prepared to experience it in graduate school. Several of my professors questioned my imagery, stating they didn't buy it. When I asked them to explain what they meant, they stated their job was to break me down and let me build myself back up. During the first year I called my husband and told him I wanted to quit, to come home. I thought to myself, "Why am I doing this? To what end?" I know now how important this questioning was, and my fear and insecurity would eventually pass. Coming from a town of 3,000 to a university campus of 45,000 was often paralyzing. Shaun counseled me to stay, and I thankfully did. I grew a thick skin and learned to articulate my art, found a like-minded group of friends and continued to build on my work. The experience of graduate school was crucial: I learned so much about being an artist and what I wanted to do with my work. The distance and separation from my family, community, and the land helped me to understand the sacred connection to the place and people of Nome, and upon completion in 1998 I went home.

Back in Nome I started a job at Sitnasuak Native Corporation. One aspect of my job was running the Sitnasuak Native Corporation Gallery. I loved it. Nome is situated on the Seward Peninsula and is a hub community for the surrounding villages.

Running this gallery, I had the wonderful opportunity of meeting and working with other artists from the Bering Straits region. Nome and the surrounding area have a history of the largest concentration of walrus ivory and whale bone carvers in Alaska. We started documenting their work, interviewing them and assisting with professional development, including resume and artist statements. It was an exciting time. While I remained in Nome, my husband worked remotely as a department of transportation construction inspector.

On May 14, 1998, my life was changed: Shaun was a passenger in a plane wreck. For three hours I anxiously awaited his fate. All nine people survived the crash into Newton Mountain, and I told him I wanted to move to an area where he didn't have to commute to his job by plane. Almost losing him was a wake-up call; all the small stuff fell away, another moment of clarity.

After the plane wreck I moved to Fairbanks while Shaun continued to work remotely outside of Nome. I took a position as an adjunct professor at the University of Alaska Fairbanks, which was gratifying in many ways but was also demanding and financially trying: I made more income as an instructor in graduate school. Shaun then transferred to Anchorage, and we bought our first home. I took a position as a program manager at the Alaska Native Heritage Center. It was very rewarding, and I stayed there for several years. I continued to make artwork and found myself inspired by the other Alaska Native artists I was surrounded by in my day job. I made small handmade objects throughout my youth, and as gifts for friends and family as an adult, but I had never considered it for income. People began special ordering my work. I started hosting an artist group that came together to sew, bead, eat, laugh, and enjoy each other's company. Still today I have a group of friends that come together from time to time: sometimes to work on large-scale installations or to help prep for jewelry orders, other times just for a glass of wine, food, and to catch up. It is lovingly called Sonya's Sweat Shop.

In 2002, I made the decision to concentrate on my art full-time and left my position at the Alaska Native Heritage Center. I had been considering it for several years before I began calculating the income I was making from art. My husband and I had a long talk about the pros and cons, and I set up a studio practice full time: it is one of the best things I've ever done. Although it was hard to give up the security of a steady paycheck, I was determined to make it work. One important facet of being self-employed was setting a minimum yearly income: some years I barely make that number, and others I double it. It is important for me to have this and other goals that keep me moving forward.

Over past years most of my income has been generated by small work sales, jewelry, and wearable art sold at art fairs/markets and wholesale through galleries and gift shops. Although I don't exhibit these works in the same way as the others, they definitely influence one another. Often I will use a shape or form in a large-scale installation that creeps into my earring or pendant designs, or material used in smaller works becomes central in bigger pieces. I like the blurred line that occurs between both. I am inspired by the relationship of our ancestors to their environment—how they used skin, fur, and membrane in material culture. It is these materials that help ground me: gathering and processing is a part of my creative practice.

Vital to me is family and community, and at the heart of this is the natural world. I love being with other people whether it be sewing and beading, grassroots gatherings, or subsistence activities like harvesting and smoking salmon. These activities fuel all of our lives, connect people and resources, and share our love for each other and this place. My desire to connect people has found me at the helm of a number of different groups, not necessarily running them, but in a start-up or advisory capacity. I consider this work to be just as important as the physical creation of my art. I am inspired by the outcomes and journey of this public engagement—it is truly moving. One example of this is working with the Alaska Native Arts Foundation (ANAF), which was in existence for 10 years. In 2002, I was a founding board member. It was created to help Alaska Native artists sell and market their art, offered grants and professional development opportunities, and gave them a place to have solo exhibitions. Today, I am happy to see the contributions from many of our artists who started their artist journey through ANAF.

My passion for connecting and activating community has allowed me to forge friendships in Alaska, across the United States, and abroad. Through conversations, exhibitions, and curation, I have been fortunate to foster gatherings on topics close to my heart. Indigenous and minority concerns are key in these talks. Through work with the Anchorage Museum and other partners, I have been able to bring some of these topics to the public: issues of food sovereignty and security, exhibiting culture, commodification of culture, and social ills of colonization and identity politics, just to name a few. Although these events take time away from my practice, I feel energized in creating opportunities for dialogue and understanding and for helping others.

I truly believe that the relationships I have made through community outreach have helped my career. As a result of my commitment to building relationships and to supporting and creating opportunities for others, I have been invited to participate in panels, lectures, committees, boards, and exhibitions. Many address the history, culture, family, and life of Northern Indigenous peoples; they also speak about the abuse, marginalization, and struggles of Indigenous peoples. Two important exhibitions addressing these issues included my work. The national traveling exhibition *Changing Hands Art Without Reservation* (2006) was one of three surveying contemporary Native American Art and locations included the Museum of Arts and Design, New York. It was an amazing experience that allowed me not only to share my work with a much wider audience but also to meet other Native American artists and scholars. Many of them have become lifelong friends. The second exhibition was *SITElines*: *much wider than a line* at the SITE Santa Fe Biennial, 2016. I was and am so honored to be included in these and other exciting exhibitions, which have allowed me to voice issues ever so present in the lives of Alaskans.

There have been many years when I have thought to myself, "Maybe you should get another job." It was during these hard times and through reflection that clarity came to me. Many of what I consider "break through" pieces often come from this kind of clarity. Then, sometime later when I have the resources to focus on work, I realize how lucky I am.

In my professional career I feel honored to have received a number of important fellowships and awards. These have allowed me in past years to create work unencumbered by financial constraints. I am blessed to have had the support of many organizations over the years. Some helped me to build a 1000-square-foot studio, and some allowed me to participate in group and solo exhibitions around North America and across the Atlantic.

I live and work in Anchorage, Alaska, with my husband, three dogs and a studio in the backyard. It is a great existence balancing life in a modern world but still listening and living the cultural traditions and values of my peoples, which include respect of land, animals, sea, and each other. I strive to do work that addresses these ideas. Every day I am thankful for the friends and family who support me to be able to share my love for Alaska and its people and to create a sense of place. *Quyana*—Thank you. ●

# SQUEAK CARNWATH

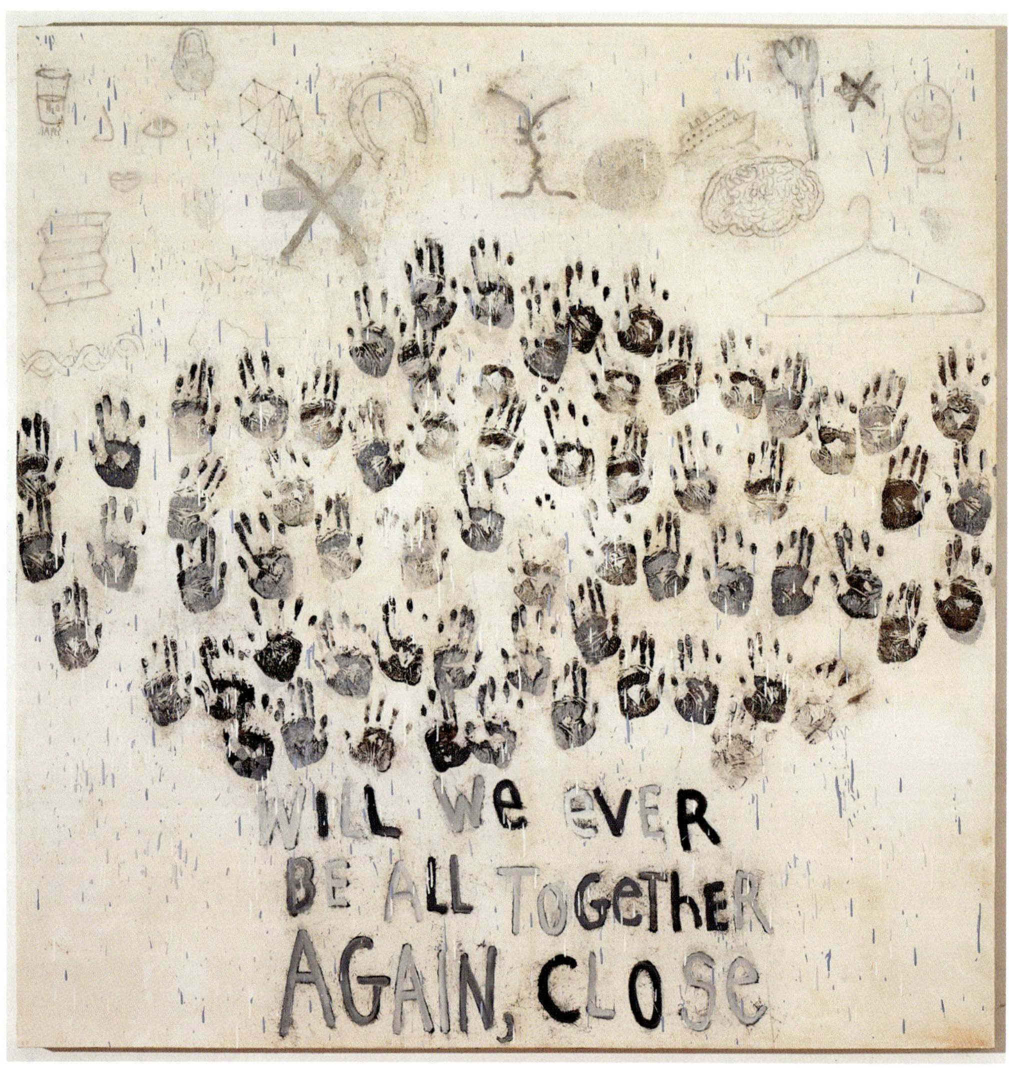

I WILL START when I left home in 1966 to go to Monticello College in Alton, Illinois, a two-year college. I majored in art and after finishing, I applied to colleges to transfer to. I was accepted at Goddard College in Plainfield, Vermont, in 1968.

I planned to spend the summer between Monticello College and Goddard at a summer program I knew about in Paros, Greece. I applied and got accepted to the Aegean Center for the Fine Arts, a program run by Tyler School of Art. This was in 1968 when I met Gary, who would become my husband five years later. He was on the island of Paros with plans to spend the rest of his life there. F ortunately, he had been rejected by the military, which was drafting young men for the war in Vietnam.

Three days after we met, we moved in together and planned to stay on the island after the summer session was over.

Squeak Carnwath
*Again*
2020
77″x77″
Oil and alkyd on canvas over panel
Courtesy of the artist and Jane Lombard Gallery, New York, NY
Photography by M. Lee Fatherree

I wrote to my parents to tell them of my plans. My mother wrote back to me about a month later. Her letter was in two parts mailed in two separate envelopes. I got part two first. She was asking me to come home because my father had started drinking again after seven years of sobriety. I should have said no.

A few weeks later Gary and I drove to Brussels, so that I could fly back home. When I got home, I realized that there was nothing I could do to fix or help my father or my mother for that matter. They needed to take care of their own problems. This was a revelation for me. I called Goddard and let them know that I wanted to attend even though I had canceled earlier that summer.

Gary came back from Europe later that fall. The following semester we were both enrolled at Goddard.

We stayed for another semester until I decided I wanted to go to art school at California College of Arts and Crafts (CCAC). I grew up on the East Coast and wanted to get as far away from what I knew to a new place. Gary was from California so he was glad to go back home. I was in school at CCAC from 1970–71 studying painting and ceramics. I dropped out three credits short of graduating. I did not see any value to having a BFA, since there were no jobs which required one.

In the next few years, we bought a house (Gary had money for a down payment; the house was $30,000 and owner financed), lived in a commune, and sold the house for a profit. I sold ceramics, worked odd jobs, and in 1975 I applied to graduate school.

I went to CCAC to speak with Viola Frey who had been my ceramics teacher when I was an undergraduate student. I had also worked in the kiln room loading kilns right after I dropped out of school but quit the job a few years earlier. I asked Viola if I applied to school in the ceramics department would she let me in. I explained that I did not want to waste the $25 application fee if I would not get accepted. Viola and the other ceramic faculty agreed to accept me into the program. In 1975 Viola could waive the three credits and let me attend without finishing an undergraduate degree (something no school today would allow). When I dropped out of California College of Arts and Crafts, I was told that without an undergraduate degree I wouldn't be able to go to graduate school by the graduate counselors. But I believed that life experience and a portfolio would count more than a BFA.

I spent the summer before graduate school sanding floors, stripping woodwork of paint, demolishing false ceilings, and taking down walls in a Victorian house (also owner financed) we bought with some of the money from the first house we sold.

Gary continued to work as a car mechanic in a shop he owned with three other men. When I was midway through graduate school at CCAC, Gary decided to go back to Berkeley to finish his degree and go on to graduate school. In 1975–77, tuition was not outrageously expensive as it is today. Both of us got some scholarship money and we had money from the sale of the house we could fall back on. As I recall, I think my tuition was only $1,200 dollars a semester, and I paid less because I got a few hundred dollars every semester from the ceramics department.

In graduate school, I worked with artists who taught at CCAC, which included Viola Frey, Jay DeFeo, and Dennis Leon. I worked in the sculpture, painting, and ceramics departments. I essentially built my own interdisciplinary major.

Even though I didn't have an undergraduate degree, I got my MFA and was able to apply for college and university teaching jobs. All of which required the terminal degree or an MFA. Thank you, Viola!

Before I got a teaching job, I worked in the ceramics department at CCAC as the "shop master" firing kilns, cleaning kiln shelves, mixing glazes, fixing kilns, hauling around 50-pound sacks of glaze material, and ordering supplies.

I rented a studio and took Polaroids of the pieces I was working on, which I propped up on my desk in the ceramics department so that I could be thinking about what I wanted to do next when I got back to the studio. When Proposition 13 passed in California, lowering property taxes, my landlord at the studio lowered my rent. Later on I would be able to follow his example.

Soon after Gary graduated, we sold the Victorian house and made a profit. We paid off our debts and banked the rest of the money.

For the next couple of years, we rented live-work spaces to see if that is what we wanted to do next instead of another house.

I continued to work in the ceramics department, teaching a little, and painting in my studio. I had time to paint because the job was only three days a week. It was a great job because I had the time to think about my work. It was, after all, a grunt job. Physical labor is a great way to get the brain going.

Between 1975 and 1980, I had a few shows, my work was in some group shows, and I won a Society for Encouragement of

Contemporary Art (SECA) award. The work was shown at the San Francisco Museum of Modern Art. In 1982, I applied for and received a Visual Artist Fellowship grant from the National Endowment for the Arts. And I started showing my work. First at Leah Levy Gallery and then at Hansen Fuller Gallery, both in San Francisco. The first show I had was at the Richmond Art Center in Richmond, California. I called and made an appointment and showed the curator my work and was invited to show it a few months later.

My first gallery show was at Leah Levy Gallery in San Francisco. She heard about my work from Lee Fatherree, who photographed my work and still does so to this day. The Leah Levy Gallery was in an apartment and not in the downtown locations with other San Francisco galleries, and after the SECA show I thought that I would leave Leah Levy Gallery and see what would happen.

In 1982, Robert Arneson mentioned my work to Hansen Fuller Gallery, where he showed. Dorothy Goldeen, an associate director, came to see the work and then Diana Fuller came to see it. They took fifteen, maybe twenty works, all about 30 × 30 inches, and filled a wall in the gallery. I asked them about representation when they had the work in the gallery. They never really answered. But I figured that with this much work on their walls, people would assume that I would show there. So it didn't matter if they represented me. They sold work and I was with the gallery for eight years. The gallery took on new partners and became Fuller Gross Gallery. I left in 1989 and began showing with John Berggruen Gallery.

In 1982, Joan Brown called me and asked me to apply for a sabbatical replacement position at UC Berkeley. She told me that she would advocate for me if I applied. Joan had seen my work at Hansen Fuller Gallery where she also showed her work. I got the job and started teaching at Berkeley in the fall. After my year of teaching at Berkeley, I got a temporary job at University of California Davis.

During the following year I applied for a tenure track position at Davis. In 1983 I joined the faculty there. Teaching gave me financial security and a chance to share information. I also learned about painting techniques that were never taught to me and showed students how to do them.

I brought paints to class so that students could try out colors they would never buy because they were on such tight budgets. In every painting class I taught, there was a rolling cart with art supplies so that students could experiment and supplement supplies they might not have.

Teaching gave me financial stability and the freedom to do what I wanted in the studio.

In 1989, my husband Gary and I bought a 21,000-square-foot warehouse building for $540,000 (which to us was a huge amount of money) with the money we had banked from the sale of the Victorian house. We only had the down payment. The building is a beautiful two-story warehouse in downtown Oakland. Again the property was owner financed. A bank never would have lent to us for a commercial building. We were young and stupid. We had no plans other than to convert it to live-work spaces for artists. We had no money to build walls, do electrical wiring, build bathrooms, put in heat, etc. Our first plan was to throw a party and invite all the artists we knew to come look at the building. We drew floor plans on the actual floor so people could see where the spaces could be. We told people that it would be a limited equity co-op so that artists would always have an affordable space to buy when owners moved or sold their units. Limited equity co-ops are set up so that the owners of the co-op do not use the property as investment or real estate speculation. No one was interested. Everyone we spoke to wanted their space to be their main investment. With the failure of that plan, we needed to figure something else out. A woman we met through a friend of ours said she was interested in becoming the developer of the building to convert to condos. She paid the mortgage for three months while we all investigated the possibility of turning the building into condominiums for artists with about six units.

Finally, we were ready to wrap up the deal, we went to her lawyers and read the contract. In the contract was a clause that stated that the building would only be rented to artists with the promise that they could purchase the space in about five years. But if the land became more valuable within that time, that they would have the right to sell the building for the land and tear it down. I got up and walked out saying that I could not do that to artists. So we ended up slowly developing the building ourselves. And we still rent to artists below market. And the spaces are large enough to work in. There are no small 300-square-foot spaces. We traded art for skylights, I got grants, and one time a dealer bought all my work for the show she wanted to have. The art dealer came to visit my studio and said she wanted to have a show of my work. I said I was booked up and on schedule to have an exhibit in San Francisco. But then a light bulb went off in my head. I saw all the sheet rock we needed along with other construction projects. And I said, "Well, if you wanted to buy the work outright I could do that because we need sheetrock." She took out her checkbook and paid for the work on the spot.

We continue to rent below market because I believe that we do not want to pay off our mortgage on the backs of artists, since we end up with the equity. We installed solar panels on the roof in 2018 which lowers the cost of electricity for us and our tenants.

Recently, I developed an exhibition space to show the work of artists in the community. Actually, the two spaces are really windows, a little like storefront windows without a store. One of them is a large box-like structure with lights and plywood beneath the sheetrock, big enough to do installations or hang a large painting. Both of the window spaces enliven the streetscape where I live and work. Now people have something to look at instead of the closed rollup doors of the warehouse. My studio manager handles the requests and applications to show and has also built websites for some of the artists. This is my stealth philanthropy. My studio manager gets paid and the artists get help and a place to show their work. We have also printed a catalogue of the first five years of the project. The catalogue, called the *EARLY YEARS* will be given to the artists and they can order more to use to promote their work and show friends. Also we maintain a website for what we call the Roll Up Project.

In 1999, I left UC Davis to go teach at Berkeley. The art department at Davis had changed and I wanted to shorten my commute. I could ride my bike to Berkeley, whereas going to

Davis was an hour-and-ten-minute drive. Wendy Sussman, a friend of mine who taught at Berkeley, wanted me to transfer to Berkeley. This is not done in the University of California system. The former chair of the Davis art department took a job in administration in the chancellor's office. He and the chair of Berkeley's art department worked out a plan. I would quit Davis one day and get hired the next day at Berkeley. This meant there would be no break in service but I would not have tenure. I was hired at Berkeley as a professor-in-residence, an appointment for tenured professors, and I remained in the UC system.

The real reason I was able to switch teaching at Davis to Berkeley is the plates Viola gave me—Wedgwood blue and white plates with images of buildings on the Berkeley campus, not unlike blue willow ware. When Viola would come over to dinner or whenever we had a dinner party, everyone was asked to pick up their plate and rub it, saying, "Berkeley, Berkeley, Berkeley" before the food went onto the plates. We carried out the ritual for about three years. And I believe it worked.

After five years at Berkeley, I got tenure. I taught at Berkeley until 2010 when I retired. After 28 years in the UC system I receive a pension, smaller than most UC professors as I reduced my teaching schedule to be less than full-time. Still, the pension helps immensely along with social security, money I have saved (especially from sales of paintings in the 1980s and 1990s).

In 2000, I wanted to start a foundation to ensure that my work would not end up on top of a garbage heap. And which would steward the work as well as give cash awards to artists. I was told by many people that I needed millions of dollars to create a foundation. I did not nor do I have millions of dollars. A lawyer I know told me that I did not need millions of dollars and that he would trade the work of setting it up for a painting of mine. When we got close to finishing the paperwork to file with the Internal Revenue Service, I told my friend Viola Frey about it. She immediately asked "can I be a part of it?" I quickly saw the value of having a foundation which could be made up of a group of artists who could pool their resources. Also I realized I did not need to have a foundation named after me or my husband. This is how the Artists' Legacy Foundation came into being. Viola died in 2004 and she became the first Legacy Artist. As the foundation's first test case, Viola's work has been catalogued, much of it documented (Viola did not document her work), exhibitions planned and executed, and because of Viola's bequest of $3 million, the foundation is able to give an annual award to an accomplished painter or sculptor, as well as steward and study the work of Viola Frey.

Legacy and care of an artists' work has been one of my favorite topics to discuss in the last few years. I realize there is a huge need for artists to think about what they want to have happen to their work. My belief is that the American visual culture must be preserved. The history of American art is not being written by only three or four well known artists. Even though at this time, in 2023, the marketplace is steering it that way.

I believe that artists have two responsibilities. The first is to give back in some way. Being an artist is an enormous privilege no matter how much money we have or don't have. We get to make our own world visible and share it with others.

And second, as artists, we need to take care of the work we make. We need to make sure that our artwork does not get lost or forgotten. This is particularly important because like America, the artwork is diverse and the artists are a diverse mirror of the population. Even if our work does not get shown over our lifetime, it is an important contribution to the visual culture of America and the world. Our artwork is a document of our time spent on the planet and that is important. We must contribute to the larger human story, so we need to make plans for what we want to have happen to our work when we are no longer here.

And now that I am 75, I want to make sure that I can paint the paintings I want to make and that our voices, artists' voices, our stories, continue to be heard and told. ●

# STEVE LOCKE

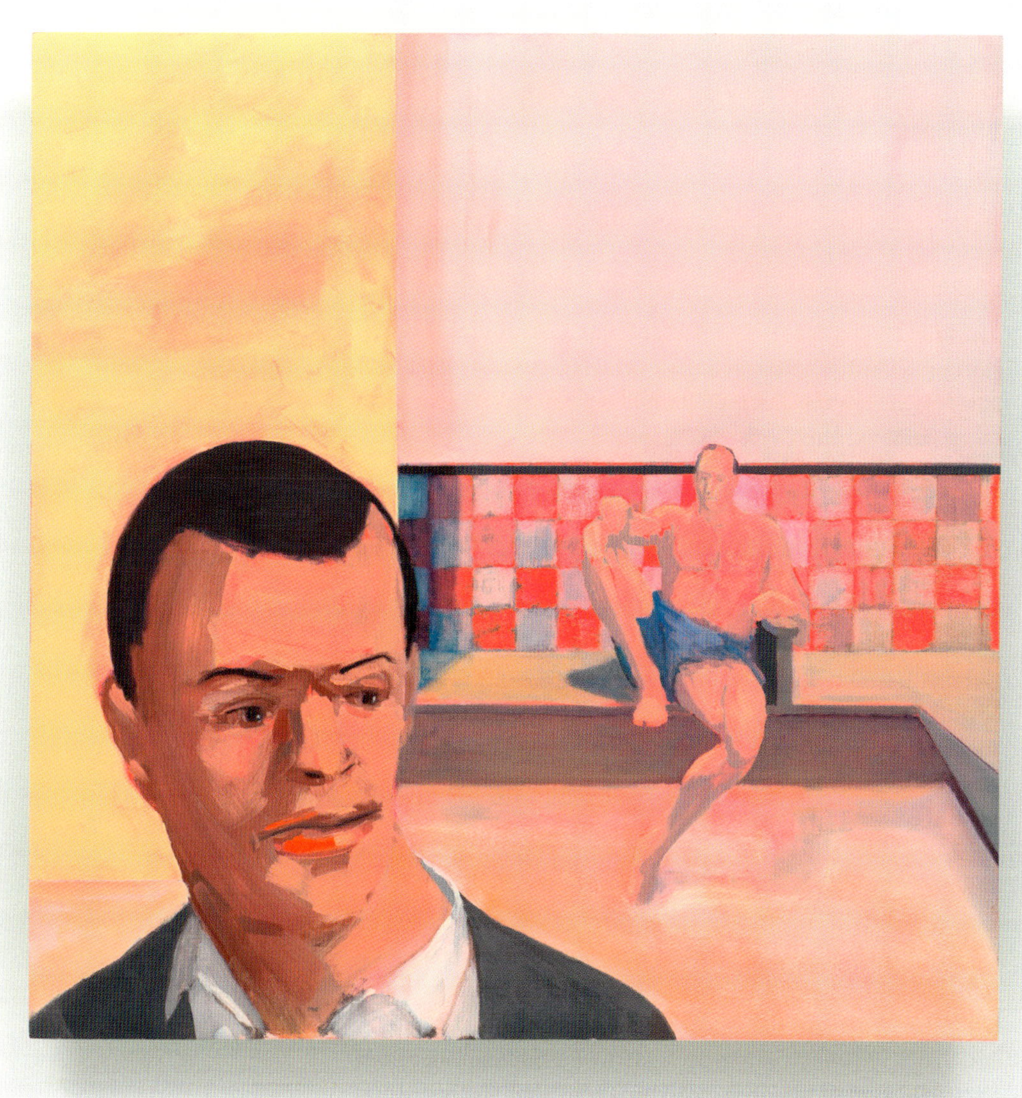

IT IS INTERESTING to me to think of myself as the last standing. I never really thought about it until I was asked to share some writing with you. Longevity is not guaranteed. I don't really think of myself as resourceful or resilient. Most days I think I am just too stubborn and too stupid to quit.

I do not come from a family of artists; my father was an autoworker; my mother was a Medicare billing clerk. Both are dead now—my father since I was a child.

I did not have the prettiest childhood and even now it is difficult for me to think too much about that time. Suffice it to say that it was brutal and lonely. And no, art was not a solace to me then. Nor is it now.

I think I really started thinking about art as something I could do when I got to Boston University in the 1980s. There was an exciting scene in Boston then around music and the visual arts. A lot of really amazing people were around. There were clubs like Spit, the Metro, Man Ray, and the 1270 that had a lot of gay and lesbian people (I don't think we called ourselves queer yet) driving what was happening in nightlife. I met artists for the first time. Real artists with studios who made stuff and talked about art. People would sit in the back room at the Ideal Diner or in Pizza Pad in Kenmore Square talking about films and bands and other artists. It was a permeable scene. I was not an artist. I went to all the parties and met the people. I was amazed by them all.

Steve Locke
*Break*
2007
23″x23″x3/4″ / 58.4x58.4x1.9cm
Oil on beveled panel

Courtesy of Alexander Gray Associates, New York
Photography by Dan Bradica

AIDS happened. All that stuff disappeared for the most part or was so decimated that it could not continue. People I loved got sick and died. People I could not stand got sick and died. Lesbians quit their jobs and became nurses to take care of men. Everything sort of collapsed. Everyone's focus was on death. I cannot really explain those days. I learned how to clean the shunt in my roommate's chest. I remember how happy me and my friends were when our friend Tom got a Hickman catheter so he would not suffer so much when getting injections. I remember so many "Celebrations of Life" for people in their twenties and thirties. I was 29. I had spent a lot of time caring for and losing lovers, tricks, friends, and colleagues. I was not the best at dealing with the immense grief and trauma that befell a lot of us during that horrible time. I went into therapy and stopped drinking in 1987.

When my closest friend John Kelley died in 1992 in Provincetown, it felt like the end of something. I was working for an insurance company as a settlement analyst. I was not moving forward or backward. I think I was just really scared to do anything. But then John died like I said, for some reason, it just felt like the end. Maybe since the worst things had already happened, there was really no reason to be scared of anything anymore. I am not certain. At any rate, that was when I decided to go to art school.

I cashed out my 401(k) to pay for the first year of school. I went to Massachusetts College of Art and Design. I worked full time at the insurance company—as a secretary instead of an analyst—to pay for the rest of it. I started over from the beginning, getting a BFA in 1997 and then getting my MFA degree in 2001. I received a full scholarship for my MFA study and worked full time while I was in my full-residency-MFA program. In 2002 I went to the Skowhegan School of Painting and Sculpture. My faculty included Robert Storr, Betty Woodman, Geoffrey Hendricks, Whitfield Lovell, and Tania Bruguera. I heard so much and learned so much in those 9 weeks. I remember Whitfield telling me to have the guts to use my own body in my work. I remember Rob telling me that there was no shame in having a job to fund your studio.

I remember Tania telling me to pay attention to the moments where something ends. I remember Geoffrey explaining how life affirming eroticism could be. I remember Betty telling me about the importance of color over shape.

Geoffrey and Betty are gone now. I miss them so.

I mark that residency as the end of my education.

I have never stopped working. I have never had a slump. I have never not known what to do. I know other artists have struggled with this and I am truly fortunate that has never been a problem.

I also have had a job. For a long time as a secretary and then finally as a professor at an art school. I love my students. I had to work hard to learn how to teach. So many people do not know how to deliver a lesson or to transmit knowledge. Teaching is not something everyone can do and it really is not the solution to artists supporting themselves. You have to love learning and you have to love the students. If you do not, then it is really hard to create the necessary environment for learning to take place. I am not referring to love in a paternalistic way or in a parental or affectionate way. When I say love, I mean the distinct feeling that one has for someone whose life can be altered by your presence. When you realize the impact a teacher has, you shift the way you engage your students. You are the model for them. You are further ahead on the path they seek. With any luck, they will surpass you and go on to teach others. Seeing them achieve and reach heights I never could is deeply inspiring.

The flip side of teaching is that it can be consuming and will devour my studio practice if I let it. I am asked constantly to do more work, more meetings, more administration, things that take me out of the class room I love. The fact that artists are terrific managers is not lost on a lot of academia. I keep declining administrative positions that would take me away from working with artists. Working with other artists is a profound privilege.

I have a simple motto: work hard; expect nothing.

I never expected anyone ever to be remotely interested in anything I did as an artist. I made my work because it was the work I believed needed to be made. Because I had a job and I could pay for my own work, I never had to worry about selling it. This allowed me to develop my own ideas and my own vision, and to keep working no matter what happened with shows of sales or any of that stuff. I stayed engaged in the artworld and went to all the openings and then went back to look at the shows. I saw/see a lot of stuff that simply pisses me off. When this happens I go back to the studio and try to make something that affirms what I think is right or true. The only solution to someone's bad work is to make good work of your own.

I was often the only black person or the only queer person in a situation. I had gallery directors do studio visits with me and ask me all sorts of awful questions like, "Why do you only paint white people?" and "Do you make any work that I can sell?" and "You don't sound black." I remember people calling me specifically in February for group shows but never being interested in me for solo projects or exhibitions. Here is the thing: I KNEW that was the way the world was. I never expected anyone in the dominant culture to love me, accept me, be happy to see me, or understand my work. People acting like you don't belong doesn't make it true. The artworld is my world too, after all, and I am not about to let people exclude me or to take on their contempt. After watching so many people die simply because they were gay I knew better than to expect anything from the dominant culture when it came to my life and my happiness. I knew it was going to be a fight for my entire life and that was just the way it was. I had to stand my ground all the time and sometimes that meant telling people that they had to leave my studio. I could not complain about what had happened because no one would have cared. The only thing I could do was work and to make the best work I possibly could. I read about art and learned how to write about art so I could create texts about my own work so I did not have to cede the narrative about my work to others.

There is some wider interest in my work now and for that I am deeply grateful. As I said, I never expected it but it is good to know that there are people who see what I am doing and are engaged in a way that is critical and passionate. •

# SUSAN LUSS

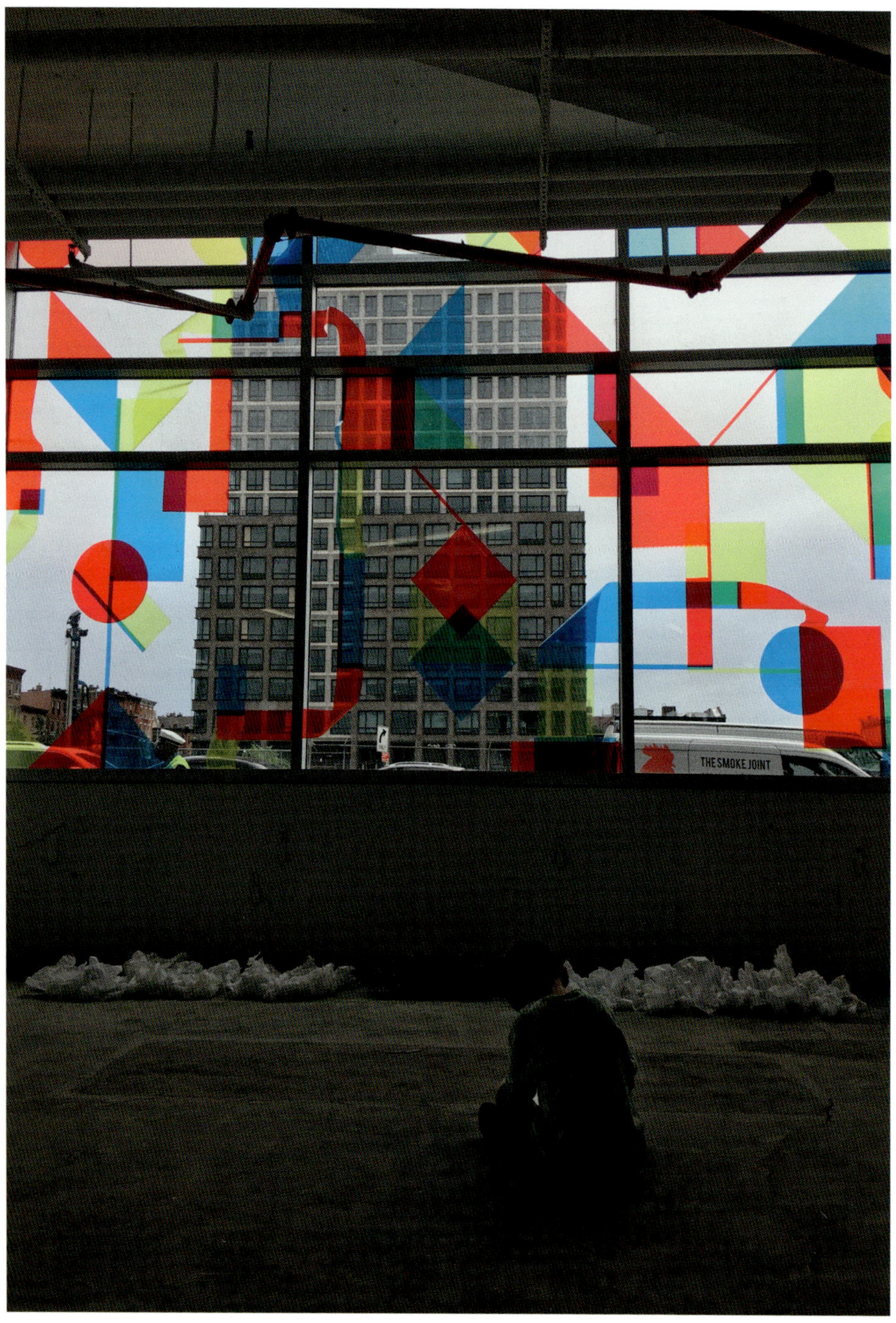

IT WAS FRESHMAN year. I remember sitting in second semester English class at Pratt Institute in Brooklyn, New York. The seats form a bow shape around the professor's desk to facilitate conversation. On one hand, I am comfortable in this environment and on the other hand, I feel like a fish out of water, hearing concepts and words whose meanings I do not know. We discuss writing devices used to develop poetry; one concept is metaphor. I had heard the word with no idea of its actual meaning, much less how to use it as a writing device. I look around wondering if I am the only student who does not know what it means, so I raise my hand and ask: what is a metaphor? That was January 2010. I was 50 years old.

Growing up in Huntsville, Alabama, back in the mid-1960s to late 1970s, I never imagined being an artist, much less starting college at age 50. My parents divorced in 1965 when I was five years old; it was a terrible rupture for me and I suffered what I call a psychic death, turning inward. Over the next twelve years living with my mom, who worked to support us, my dad being in and out of the picture, we moved eight times. It was a destabilizing and insecure period, but I had a lot of independence and took refuge being outside, where I felt safe. While I have no memory of physically moving from place to place, I do have vivid memories of the neighborhood landscapes. Those early years had a formidable impact across my entire life, sowing the seeds of my survivalist skills and resiliency born out of adversity.

Susan Luss
*Windows Pipes and Tissues*
2017
120″x216″ (site specific installation)
Architectural gels, tape
Courtesy of the artist

At age 15, I started my first job and work became the place where I felt acknowledged and valued; it was stable, and I had security. Recounting this now, it felt like a family unit. Then at 18, I moved to San Diego, California, to be with a friend. While living in San Diego I worked in retail clothing followed by four years as a member of the United Food and Commercial Workers Union, working in the grocery business, starting as a grocery bagger, then promoted fast to a check-out clerk, and later working night crew stocking shelves. It was a great job, empowering new skill development, engaging my innate aptitudes, and working with people who are still my friends today. In 1981, I left the grocery business, sold my car for money I needed to move, and headed to Hawaii where my mother lived. There I lived independently, supporting myself working in a retail clothing store. In 1983, I met a young man from New York who was vacationing in Hawaii with his family. After a brief time together, he asked me to come live with him in Brooklyn. I moved to New York in June and soon thereafter started work full time in the garment industry, which provided financial security and the opportunity to engage and work with people from all walks of life. We married in 1988 and in 1991 we bought a house and moved to Long Island. I continued working in the garment industry but by 1996 was deeply unfulfilled, leading me to question the purpose of my life. At the time I felt desperate to get out of what was inside me, even though I had no idea what it was I would "get out."

That winter, I remember standing in a field late afternoon, and listening to wind rustle bare branches, thinking if I could learn to paint maybe then I could "get out" of me what felt unspeakable. Painting seemed a form of communication, of pure language. It was not about art or being an artist. Four years went by and in March 2000 I summoned the courage to leave my job in the garment industry. A month later, my husband was diagnosed with metastatic melanoma cancer. Over the next three years, while going through many rounds of treatment, he continued working and I started a new career as a business development manager in contract office furniture, marketing the services of the company through creating and sustaining professional relationships across diverse industries. Between his cancer diagnosis in 2000 and his death in February 2003, we lived as best we could under the circumstances. On my own, I gave myself over to grief so raw all I could do was accept it flowing through and transforming me.

Out of necessity, I continued working as a business development manager in contract furniture. In May 2003 a professional colleague, Michael Spector, knowing of my recent loss, suggested an introduction to Gerald Luss, director of facility design for North Shore LIJ Hospital system (now Northwell Health). Michael wanted to help me professionally, knowing the introduction could be instrumental in awarding my company business. Michael made an appointment for us to meet with Gerald on May 30, 2003, at 10:00 a.m. Entering Gerald's office I saw the back of his head and he stated, "I will be right with you." A bright surge of energy flooded my body. I do not know how else to describe it. What was supposed to be a five-minute meeting lasted two hours. In retrospect, I understand my capacity to grieve so deeply the recent loss I suffered created a place in my soul that Gerald inhabited from that moment, and we have been together ever since. I was 44; he was 78.

As our lives intertwined, we commuted between his apartment in Manhattan and my house in Greenvale on Long Island, New York. In January 2004, while on a brief family leave from my job, I started taking painting lessons at The Stevenson Academy, a small local art school in Oyster Bay, Long Island. The moment I picked up a paint brush I remembered that day in 1996 when I imagined painting could be a form of language. That July, Gerald and I married, combining our homes to live at his apartment in the city and I transferred to my company's office in Manhattan.

Over the next few years, I continued working part time, contributing financially to our household. During these years I learned more about Gerald's long and impactful career as an architect, which began as he left Pratt Institute in 1949. Gerald's historical relationship with Pratt led me to enroll there in 2008 for classes in drawing and painting, subsequently applying to matriculate in the bachelor's program starting fall semester of

2009, which meant I had to quit my job. During the months-long decision-making process, I understood for the first time that my identity, my entire sense of self-worth, had been attached to my jobs for over 35 years, and I was walking away from that. The process helped me question who I could be without those attachments. It felt like going back in time, re-experiencing all those years of disruptive movement beyond my control as a child. It was scary. On the flip side I gained clarity through understanding the importance, the absolute value, of the years I sustained myself and others through the work of building meaningful relationships with people from all over the world. They were my family. I loved working and took great pride in what I had accomplished. While I felt extreme discomfort about the cost of a four-year education, Gerald was my biggest supporter, both emotionally and pragmatically. Between all my years working and saving and Gerald's ongoing architecture practice, he helped me gain confidence in my decision to go to college full time.

While at Pratt, besides the intrinsic value of education and a deepening awareness of the power of visual arts, I forged new and lasting relationships with fellow students and professors alike. It was similar in experience to my former work in that engagement with my colleagues was essential for sustaining life. Three months before graduation from Pratt, on the morning of February 14, 2013, a fire gutted the senior painting studios and 27 of us lost everything. The experience was traumatic for me. Three years of my work was destroyed, including all my journals and writings. But it was also transformative because I realized a kind of freedom from the loss that prepared me for new growth. Post-graduation I rented a studio in Long Island City, Queens, in New York City, which was a three-mile walk from our apartment. It was the first time in my life I had an independent place outside of home. Besides developing my own work, I used the studio for group critiques and painting sessions with my friends from Pratt. As my work evolved, I decided I wanted more dialogue to understand what was growing there. I applied to three master of fine arts programs located in New

York City. I was accepted to the School of Visual Arts (SVA) commencing September 2014.

During two years at SVA, one mentor, David Row, was a steadfast guide helping me develop insights to the questions that drove me to graduate school in the first place. He did not insist I make objects, instead engaging with what he saw in my studio: a gathering of collected material found on my daily walks to school, transforming daily as I continually added and rearranged the assemblage, and hourly as light shifted, creating new relationships. The studio had its own life, and I was an active material in the process, a kind of go-between. There were times I considered my childhood experience as relevant to the work but resisted talking about it. Nor did I want to talk about my experience with death and the lingering consequences of trauma and long-term grief. Eventually I understood speaking about these things was essential to my growth and found support among my colleagues who had the courage to talk about their own life experiences through their work.

At SVA I did not learn skills as I had at Stevenson and Pratt but realized the entirety of my life experience provided me with an inexhaustible source of material. All those years ago when I went underground to survive, that 5-year-old was alive and well at 57 and more curious than ever. The time I spent at SVA helped shift my self-perception, making way for more intentional work. I will never forget, just out of SVA, one of my former Pratt professors recommended me to a local collaborative residency. She had a sense of what life just out of graduate school could be like and wanted to support me entering the creative arts through collaborative engagement. Over the years I have realized my entire life is sustained through a diversity of relationships and experiences. These are intergenerational not only because of the relationships formed with my colleagues and professors from Pratt and SVA, but also due to relationships I developed and maintained throughout the years working in business, supporting and connecting people across industries.

Besides my studio practice and responsibilities at home, I work with the creative and academic community in a variety of ways. For example, as an active alumna of Pratt, I serve on a fine arts committee, curating exhibitions providing Pratt alumni with opportunities to exhibit. There are intermittent projects requiring specialized knowledge and skills, so I look to my network, engaging their services. I have been invited by friends in academia as a visiting artist guest speaker for their classes, be it professional practice, research, color theory, among other topics. That is one of my favorite things to do because it is direct engagement with students and sometimes leads to mentorship. But simply sharing time and space with another person in friendship, being a good listener, being present, is important to me; it's not outwardly measurable but it is mutually life sustaining.

Fast forward three years since I began this writing journey. It is the end February 2022 and much has changed across the world because of the pandemic. (And so much more that is out of the scope of this essay.) While I am back at work in the studio now, for most of 2020 it was off limits, so I started to work in the only place available that felt marginally safe apart from our home: the urban landscape. This period foregrounded aspects of my practice that had previously operated in the background. For example, using environmental forces like wind and rain as active participants in the creative process. Collaborating with the wind is powerful for me. It provides an outlet for grief that is beyond words. Also, during the early months of the pandemic, there was a reconnection process amongst some of my female friends, deepening the commitment to our collective wellbeing. We are like a forest, an alive and thriving mycorrhiza network of "mutual symbiotic association" working together, actively supporting each other across the gamut of our life's endeavors; reciprocity in action helping sustain all our lives.

The pandemic brought Gerald's and my creative lives in closer proximity because we were both working from home. I still don't know exactly how to contextualize it but there was something in the way his work designing and building timepieces and my work in response to the changing environment outside evolved during that early pandemic time that connected and overlapped. I also learned more about his desire from the age of eight to be an architect. The importance for him of designing interior space for the needs of people's lives who inhabit the space, opposed to creating a monument to oneself. Because I was creating work outside amongst the public, I was experiencing something that seemed similar. Creating a visual language that exists outside of oneself that others can experience. For me, working in real-time outside was new territory and during the early pandemic an aspect of daily life that sustained me emotionally, providing me with energy to care for both of us. And then there was all the Zooming.

Since that moment sitting in my freshman year English class at Pratt in 2009, I have come to recognize that metaphorical thinking is instinctual for me. I also appreciate that I did not imagine nor choose to be an artist when I was young but lived and worked my way toward it over a 60-plus-year lifespan. The adversity of my childhood led directly to my resiliency. The work I did through my jobs over 35 years provided not only stability and financial security but they are where I developed skills and honed my innate aptitudes essential to being a human living in the world today. I learned that death, fire, and now a pandemic, while unimaginably tragic and awful, can be freeing and transformative. Through arts education later in life I learned about the vital role artists have in the world. All those years of building a career for myself outside of the arts, learning to trust myself and others, having a loving and stable relationship with Gerald, are pillars which sustain not only my life, but are foundational to my desire in helping sustain other lives. ●

# SUSANNA COFFEY

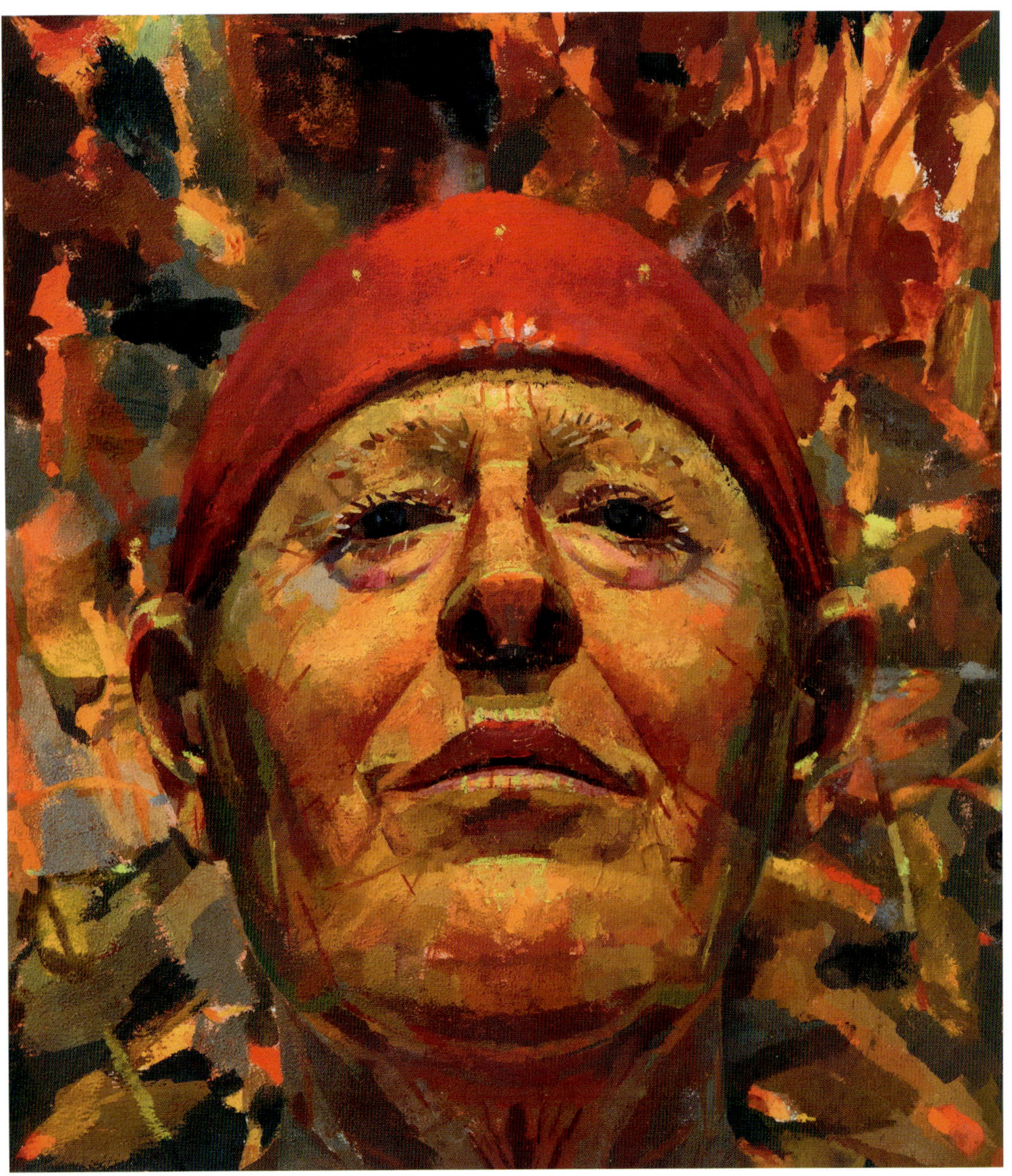

WHY AND HOW at 74 years of age am I still standing up for my art and my student's artistic future? I've been painting and drawing since I was a child, and teaching for at least 50 years so it's hard to write about all that time, all those experiences … too much information. Nothing I recount here can explain the artwork, it must speak for itself. As for teaching, the job is to shepherd students to a place where my voice will dissipate and theirs will grow strong and independent. The artist and teacher that I am is totally in love with the evolving history, craft, and materiality of painting. It lives and vibrates for me, and always has. In my own art I'm inspired to resist, compete with, and emulate traditions that began in prehistory and are morphing as we speak. In school, I seek to conserve those traditions. There will always be young artists who find that painting's language speaks to, and for, them and see that something in its history remains undone or underrepresented.

Over a lifetime an artist's life can be so joyful, rewarding, and full of surprises. There is some kind of gravitational pull among those who love culture. Happenstances that bring me to new friends, communities, and countries have been more common than not. But tragedies, struggles, ego-crushing failures, and constant self-criticism have also colored this life. All artists live under an uncertain star; there are no rules governing a career's trajectory. The only guideline we can be sure of is "do the work."

Susanna Coffey
*Video et Taceo*
2018
12″x11″
Oil on panel
Courtesy of Steven Harvey Fine Art Projects and the artist
Photography by Jenny Gorman

I don't think I've ever walked a clear, well-lighted path. What follows, in no particular order, are a few stories about my past.

Construction sites made the best of playgrounds. At 4 years old, going to work with my father, World War II veteran Edwin Coffey, was Heaven. A wild, chaotic landscape of raw material was there for me to explore. In my imagination the mud puddles, boulders, concrete blocks, culvert pipes, piles of gravel, lots of sand, and stacks of lumber would become castles, cities, or other planets. It was ok to draw on pretty much any surface I could find. We were then living in Chittenango, New York, where dad was working on the construction of the New York State Thruway; we moved a lot in the 1950s. Although I didn't know many other children, I don't remember being lonely, just busy. There were a few invisible friends to play with. Sometimes dad would take me to the jobsite garage with its huge machines, colorful bins and boxes, pencils and chalks, oily smells, tools of all kinds, and a group of mechanics who always had time for a curious, talkative little girl. According to my father and his friends, when asked "What do you want to be when you grow up?" I answered, "I want to be a master mechanic or an artist." Now 70 years later I see that I am both: a solitary, tinkering worker who maintains the tools of her trade, keeps a studio running at all costs, and creates painting after painting.

That 4-year-old who somehow knew in her bones that she was an artist had no idea about being a teacher. I hated school. My mother, Magel Willingham Coffey, a WWII combat nurse who taught her toddler to read and love books with a passion that schools seemed to disallow. Reading was a real home and haven for me. (When I visited Frida Kahlo's Blue House, on her bookshelf I saw that she too had read Dostoyevsky's *The Idiot.*) Prince Myshkin helped me endure high school. Books and stories, Miss Florence Hill read the tale of Persephone's abduction and showed her second graders a pomegranate. I then understood in a child's way that even gods can commit crimes and I should watch out for Hades and Zeus. The old stories, not so old really.

On October 27, 1954, my mother held a tiny baby up to her hospital window for me to see. There she was! She would be the writer Jane Carroll Coffey. Jane, my sister and friend who has, from the beginning, inspired, sustained, and encouraged me. While I struggled somewhat to relinquish my only-child status, the rewards of this relationship have always been immeasurable. Most of my memories are shared with her, sometimes corrected by her. As a toddler, I remember Jane, the future novelist, in her plaid overalls and cropped hair, propped up in front of our mother's old Underwood, totally absorbed, pecking away at the keys. Many days we ran wild together, with our dogs Lady and Ludwig. Over fields, making forts and igloos, we played games of the imagination. Usually, we shared a bedroom. Jane's bed was home to so many stuffed animals and dolls there was hardly room for her little self. Her ability to treat them carefully, as living things, showed me how to not lose that magical way of thinking common to most young children. Now I know she convinced me of the truth. *All beings* have a life of some kind, *natura vivat*, rather than *nature morte*. In 1969 she and her friend Joyce cajoled me to take their fourteen-year-old selves to the Woodstock Festival in my Volkswagen bus. I came back east, fearful, and under the sway of past traumas. But like she has so many times, Jane brought me into a truly wonderful experience. Those three days of rain, mud, and non-stop joyful music, the comradeship of Jane, Joyce, and those half-million other nonviolent attendees alchemically helped me out of a very dark place. She has been the best friend, the mentor, her words and actions have given me the ability and desire to continue.

At 21, I married a drummer. Sketchbooks were my only studio while we traveled for his gigs or lived in the "bandhouse." There was not much time or space for me to find my artist-self but I did hear great, great music! Nights of seeing artists like Janice Joplin, Ben E. King, Sun Ra, Flora Purim, Pharoah Sanders, Muddy Waters, Jr., and others showed me how hard and passionate a real artist works at what they do. The rock & roll housewife thing was not so great but around 1973, I read *The Second Sex* and found *Ms. Magazine*, listened to every Nina Simone record I could find, and was puzzled about how I could leave that scene and become a real artist. When we lived in Providence, Rhode Island, one February day the husband dropped me off at work, emptied our joint checking account, and left the several-months-pregnant me without a word. A late-term abortion, illness, and homelessness followed, but one step, one low-wage job at a time, I crawled back into my own life. LOL, at 24 I went to a high school for my SATs in order to apply to college.

I went to the University of Rhode Island in 1973, not as a student, but as a model for drawing classes. Years later I lectured there and the professor I had modeled for joked that he didn't recognize me with my clothes on. Modeling was a good job, I learned so much about drawing, teaching, and being still. In 1975, when I matriculated at the University of Connecticut, another professor asked me why would a woman want to be an artist when she could have babies? Seriously, Nathan Knobler? At UConn the photographer "Wild Bill" Parker took our class to a show of Bob Thompson's paintings. In those years I was told that painting was dead but Thompson's work showed me that painting is a continuum, a slipstream anyone could enter and experience time travel. I also got to study the art of West Africa under Tamara Northern, and discovered a canon of art in which human or animal imagery can be reconfigured and reinvented to reveal psychological, spiritual, political, and/or emotional states of being. But what was my path as an artist? As an undergrad I knew that I was, in my soul, a painter, a figurative painter. And that I loved painting but would always have something like Keats' Negative Capability in regards to what's missing, wrongly wrought, or propagandistic in its history.

1977 was The Year of the Snake, a poisonous year when my sister and I lost our strong, elemental, great-hearted, beloved, and loving mother to cancer. But like so many others I was driven deeper into my art by the death of the person I loved most. Images of her were what I had left and I tried to paint her back into being. 1977 was also the year a show of prehistoric figures, including the Venus of Willendorf, came to the Natural History Museum in New York. That year I also discovered the Met's Fayum encaustic portraits. The ancient objects felt (and still feel) so immediate, so alive, so resistant to death's erasures. That's my sense of beauty.

Some people get up in the morning, look in the mirror, and get ready to go to work. I'm a painter who works mostly in self-portraiture, so I get up, go to work, and then spend hours looking into a mirror. This is not the place to go on about my art, I'd rather not. But there is something about these portraits that I have never talked about. I think I spend so much time looking at my reflection in order to understand that I'm still alive and in what way. In 1967, when I was 17, I was walking from Port Authority to Penn Station. At 8th Ave and 38th street in Manhattan, I was assaulted. My attacker forced me into a parking lot, was on top of me preparing to stab me in the heart when he lost his grip, and dropped the knife right by my hand. I then stabbed him in his back, he got off me and ran away and it was over but not in the way I expected. I was so sure I would die, but then I didn't. A thread snapped. The person who poses so patiently in my studio's mirror is one that I feel I must keep track of, she makes me uneasy. I observe that face as I paint, and work on a picture for days, weeks, months, sometimes years, until the figure on my canvas feels completely and independently, alive on its own.

At 23, divorced (whew) and finally taking my art life seriously, I made some deals with myself. I was on my own and wanted to live the kind of life I have now, that of a productive, working artist and a seasoned, engaged professor. There were very few role models in those years. The how-to for a career in art or academe seemed arcane; to thrive in both … impossible.

In New Haven, Connecticut, the late-1970s recession made it possible to find a studio space, but it was hard to find a way to support it. I've had so many jobs: waitress, bartender, housecleaner, chambermaid, artist's model, nurse's aide, file clerk. But in 1977 all the jobs were scarce and I was scraping by, bussing tables. Luckily, I applied and qualified for employment under the federal Comprehensive Employment and Training Act (CETA) and was assigned to clerical work in its offices. But what I really wanted was to be assigned to one of CETA's arts programs for teens. Fortunately, the Theater Program's dance instructor quit without notice, and so I became a teacher. As the only person on staff with even a little dance experience (thanks

American Bandstand, Maximilian Froman, Alvin Ailey's kid's classes), I volunteered to step in. At that very first class, I knew a door had opened and I felt that this teaching thing was work I could do. I've never wanted children of my own, but I love working with young people.

Teaching is not exactly art, but it's close to it. That season I showed each kid how to stretch, find their best moves, and introduced them to a history that they might want to become part of. That job led to other art classes. Up to and throughout my MFA time at Yale I taught painting and drawing to at-risk youth, psych patients, and incarcerated men at the New Haven Correctional Center and others.

Living illegally (with my dog Jude) in a huge, unheated studio at 15 Orange Street in New Haven was possible because of those teaching jobs. Without hot water or a shower, I slept under a work table, made many bad paintings, met artist/musician friends (Riley Brewster, Lin Duer, Legs McNeil, Kyle Staver, The Saucers) and shared that space with a mime troupe (LOL, they were *not* quiet).

Art studios: what haven't I done for them? Living and working in deserted buildings, with drug dealers, loud, bad musicians, and angry drunken men as neighbors. 1322 S. Wabash, Chicago, Illinois, abandoned by its owner, had no heat or electricity. The stairwell to the tenth floor was totally dark, but once I was in the studio there was 4,000 square feet of light-filled space awaiting me. At 1600 S. Michigan, Chicago, I slept with my cats on an air mattress in a loft with no secure door but with windows that looked out on the old Chess Studios and from where one could watch carriage horses run freely around a vacant lot. #1 Lispenard St, New York City, was right above an all-night bar's sound system. On nearby Walker Street, there were lots of spaces without heat or light, but enough room to paint my first one-person show in 1994 at Gallery Three Zero in New York City

There were others. The worst, strangely enough, was on Lake Como in a very posh residency. It was a narrow room next to the laundry and had one small window. It had a low ceiling that couldn't fit an easel, and the floor was broken into two levels. But there I met an executor of Wittengenstein's estate, swam among schools of silver fish under the Swiss Alps, saw snakes mating in the gardens and because there was a show to make, I made do with the studio. The memories of even my most derelict studios are so fond. I remember each one like a lover with whom I lived happily and productively but eventually had to leave.

Before 1982, I had never even been to Chicago, Illinois, but that spring, in my last semester completing the MFA Program at Yale, I was hired to teach figure painting classes at The School of the Art Institute of Chicago (SAIC). Thirty-seven years later in 2017 I retired as the FH Sellers Professor in Painting.

How did I get that job? It was because I chatted with the wonderful Philip Salem outside a convenience store on York Street in New York in the summer of 1981. That July I had a work/study job on the art building's maintenance crew. On lunch breaks we'd walk down to the Wawa convenience store for coffee and snacks. There I'd see this slender silver-haired man hanging out near the store, nursing a coffee, reading and people watching. He'd flirt a little with some of the crew. With his sly smile and such bright eyes, I liked him immediately, something about him seemed special. One day I saw him reading Jean Genet's novel, *Our Lady of the Flowers*. Having just read it, I spoke with him about the book and how much I loved it. We became friends right away (I later found out he had known Genet in Europe). I learned that Philip was homeless, ate at soup kitchens, went to free concerts and movies, read library books, took long walks in the country, and lived as artful a life as he possibly could. In his youth he had danced professionally, starred in Maya Deren and Alexander Hackenschmied's short experimental film, *Meshes of the Afternoon*, drank too much, fell down in just about every way and found himself, in his 60s, living on New Haven's streets.

Soon after meeting Philip I was able to find him work modeling for artists, and of course he became popular, eventually leaving the street for his own place. One day at school while waiting for some paint to dry I rummaged around the critique space looking for something to read and I found a *New York Times Book Review*. As I thumbed through, I found a query at the bottom of one of the pages by filmmaker Jonas Mekas, asking for information about a Philip Salem whom he wanted to interview for a piece he was writing about Maya Deren! I found Philip and the next week Mekas sent a limo car to pick him up at his shelter and wined, dined, and celebrated him. I was always so happy to make his life easier but *his* help to me was so substantial, he made me change my way of thinking about the future.

It was 1981 and my idea for life after graduation was to keep my studio, paint, maybe waitress, maybe some part-time teaching... or move to Greece, or go back to Mexico. There was no plan. But Philip uncharacteristically gave me a very harsh talking-to when he heard that I wouldn't at least try to find a teaching job. He made me promise to go to the Annual College Art Association (CAA) conference in New York. Other classmates had set up interviews there, but with no resume or proper clothes to wear I thought, "why bother." Philip emphasized that I MUST seize every opportunity to secure a meaningful source of self-support as he had not. So I borrowed a tweed suit, typed a resume (so thick with Wite-Out that each page looked sculptural) and shared a hotel room with several other students. Once there I looked at the lists of schools who were interviewing anyone at all, and joined those lines, the longest of which was for SAIC. After a two-hour wait, I was interviewed by professor Tony Philips, now a dear friend. It must have gone well, because they hired me for a one-year visiting artist position (that lasted 37 years). Back in New Haven, I thanked Philip with all my heart and made an asparagus omelet for a celebratory brunch.

The next year at Christmas break, driving through a blizzard on my way back to Connecticut, a huge Snowy Owl flew straight toward my windshield, it startled me and then disappeared into the forest. I wondered if I'd get to see Philip again. When I got to New Haven friends told me he had passed away quietly, in his own apartment.

Now I still paint and draw, dance, walk the wondrous Chessie "the pup" Barker, travel to see art and artists, study with master dancers, write about other people's work, read the manuscripts of my brilliant sister, buy too many books, and adore my friends.

I'm currently making an inventory and archive of all my artwork to date, yikes. With two shows of my own work scheduled I'm also curating some shows of other artist's work. A new series of my nine woodcut prints based on the story of Demeter and Persephone has just been published by the LeRoy Neiman Center for Print Studies at Columbia University. I'm now retired from teaching but still involved with it all. Soon I'll be volunteering at the Planned Parenthood clinic up the street. I'm standing but not very still. ●

TARANEH HEMAMI

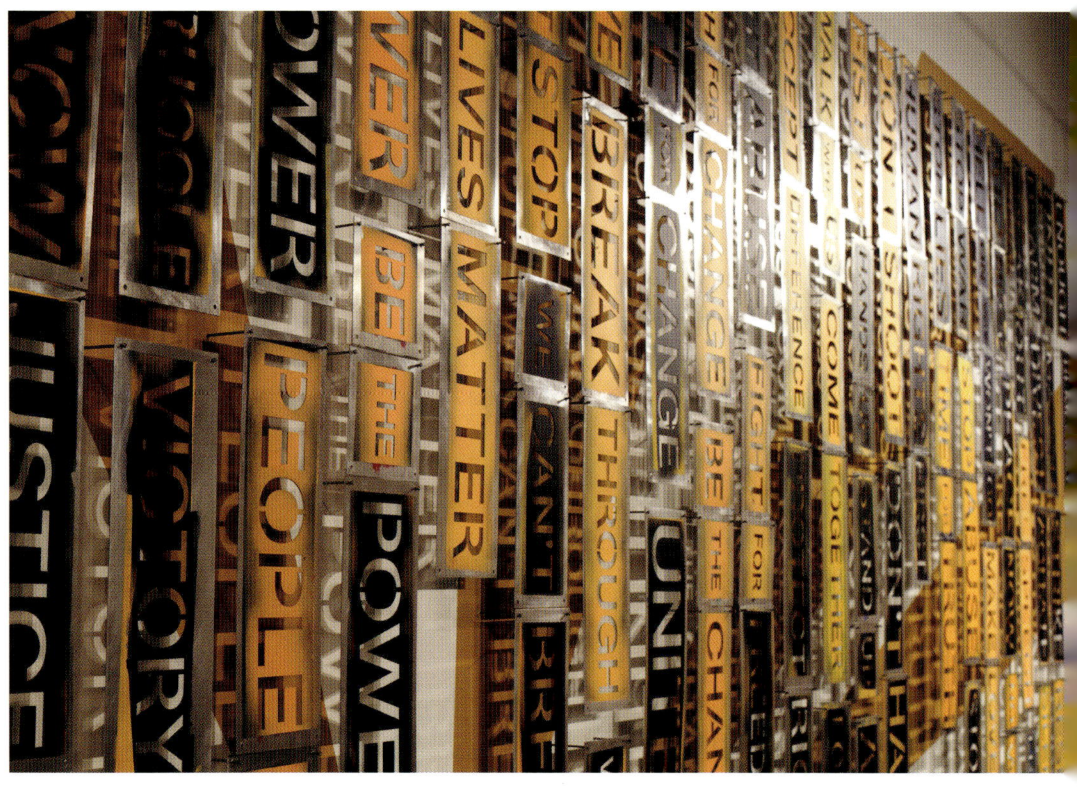

ARMED WITH THE recent edition of Haim's Persian/English dictionary in my suitcase and the Qur'an my grandma insisted for me to take on the plane as protection, I headed to the University of Missouri, in Columbia, Missouri, in January 1978 to study art for a few years and gain life experiences beyond my family's small corner near the Alborz Mountains in Northern Tehran. My dream was to devote all my efforts to perfecting my craft, believing that despite my limited training and exposure to contemporary art, my dedication and passion would carry me through to wherever I would dare to call myself an artist before returning home. It only took one semester in the harsh winter of Columbia, Missouri, to transfer to the University of Oregon, where I had a few acquaintances. It was a welcome change to be out of the dormitories, living with roommates who soon became close friends. I had found a place to settle down with a small but growing community, to learn about the people, culture, and politics of where I had landed, immersed in the lush, forever-green landscapes of Eugene, Oregon.

Political tensions were palpable in Iran beginning in January 1977 and by October 1978, rage had inflamed Iran when many demonstrators were shot dead by the regime, forever changing the course of the country's future. A revolution was about to erupt in Iran, its effects still reverberating in my world and in my works.

Taraneh Hemami
*People Power*
Since 2015
Variable installation
Aluminum, nails, acrylic, and mural on wall
Courtesy of the artist

With little understanding of the powers at play, I watched my future unfolding in two- to three- minute segments on American daily news; watching from a vast distance away from the only home I had known with much anxiety as the chants of millions of demonstrators for freedom in the streets of my childhood, changed to demands for the return of Ayatollah Khomeini. The monarchy was toppled in no time, and by spring 1979, the Islamic Republic of Iran was born, systematically wiping out any opposition with sheer force and imposing a "Cultural Revolution," while changing the system of governance inside out.

In November 1979, the U.S. Embassy in Tehran was attacked, Americans were taken hostage, turning all Iranian nationals living in the United States into suspects overnight, and in the following months thousands were deported over minor visa issues. The relationship between the United States and Iran was severed, and traveling between the two countries became impossible. My parents were no longer able to visit from Iran, and although the distance was difficult to bear, they urged us to continue with our studies in the United States and wait out these unpredictable times. It was a great sacrifice for them given the hardships they were experiencing in Iran, and the pressure of the exorbitant tuition for their three daughters studying abroad. I struggled through full loads of university requirements every semester to be able to graduate early and return home as soon as it became possible. Soon however, the invasion of the country by neighboring Iraq in the fall of 1980 ignited an eight-year war, and all our efforts shifted on getting our parents out of Iran.

Longing for home and family became a constant condition; watching my country being bombed day after day, a wrenching experience. It was comforting to be around other Iranians. Our gatherings became my refuge; it was where we learned more than what the U.S. media was reporting on Iran, exchanging stories and resources to track the continuously-changing situation. As the conflict deepened between the United States and Iran, so did the tensions within the Iranian community, and the yearly celebrations of Persian New Year Nowruz organized by the Iranians Student Association (ISA) seemed to be the one place that brought everyone together in peace. I helped with

ISA cultural programming the last few years of my studies in Eugene. Soon after graduation, most of the small community I had built dispersed, seeking work in different parts of the U.S.

I moved to the Bay Area along with a few friends in January 1982. The two-story house we rented in Daly City became a refuge to many friends and family coming for job opportunities in the newly developing Silicon Valley. It was where we gathered to cook together, share stories, and exchange political views, gradually building connections to the growing Bay Area Iranian community. It was where we planned to wait for the war to end, for the political conflicts to be settled, for the world to change.

As years went by, Iran became more distant from my everyday realities, and I became increasingly unfamiliar with the nuances impacting its continuously evolving politics. I too, was changing, learning about myself as well as the new world around me, with little prediction of what the future would hold. I became involved with the Iranian cultural organizations in Berkeley, and began attending the many lectures and performances regularly, eventually moving to the East Bay. Heated debates and continuous analysis of the political changes was increasingly common, ending life-long friendships and tearing families apart. We mourned the loss of many during the revolution, the arrests of thousands of members of the opposition groups, and the daily casualties of the ongoing war.

In the United States, with a recession in full swing, those of us with art degrees were struggling to find ways of surviving. While Silicon Valley was nurturing their future millionaires, most of the jobs I was able to find were in the service industry, living from paycheck to paycheck. Although I cherished the chance to get to know many people from all walks of life, those years remain the most difficult and anxiety-filled times in my life.

Making ends meet was challenging, and my broken English and limited knowledge of the world around me made it even more difficult. My dream of a creative path gave me determination and a purpose that motivated me to push through my financial hardship. Witnessing the brutality of war from a distance, consumed with pain and anger, my creativity was my tool for surviving these volatile years, allowing me to stay focused, driven, sane, content. I felt quite isolated, and graduate school seemed to be my only option to find my way back to my art practice and build connections to the arts community. It took several years to make ends meet, to create a strong body of work and apply for graduate school. Stephen Goldstine, the director of Graduate Studies at California College of Arts and Crafts (CCAC) encouraged me to apply for their program and continued to support my path as an artist. I still had to work full time to sustain myself, but I spent every open hour at the studios creating, while building life-long friendships. Inspired by so many brilliant faculty, I began working closely with Raymond Saunders, Dennis Leon, and Larry Sultan as well as Lynn Marie Kirby and Cariadne Margaret Mackenzie-Hooson, who have continued to be my mentors, colleagues, and friends.

I was finally able to travel to Iran in the summer of 1990, mainly to spend time with my father, the only one in my family still living in Iran. It was a moving experience for me, confusing and filled with pain and anguish. I had changed, as did the world I had left behind. Upon my return to the Bay Area, I needed more than ever to make sense of the transformative experience of exile, to try to understand the conflicting influences within me; the longing, the angst, the outrage, tenderness, and the intimacy of the spaces of belonging. Emotionally drained, I spent my last year at CCAC trying to reconcile the beauty and the weight of the dark-as-night memories through my creative process; revelations shook my core of the two disparately different worlds that impose their anxieties on my everyday existence, and in my works. Two years later, my father's sudden passing brought my entire family together to Tehran. His body, along with his many untold stories, were buried on the land he refused to leave. I poured my grief into my work in the year of mourning that followed, working with a few photographs that had remained as evidence of his life, of our home, and a country from which I had now become estranged. My work became a mirror to my journey through time, as essential as breathing, crucial to surviving these pain-filled years.

The art community in the Bay Area gave me refuge and offered opportunities that have continued to inspire and create a sense of home. My studio at the Headlands Center for the Arts after graduating, became a sanctuary (1992-95), broadening my worldview, meeting incredible local, national, and international artists. I had begun teaching art with a few educational institutions in public schools as well as learning new technologies to design websites. Trying to work part time to allow for studio time meant keeping my cost down to its bare minimum. Priced out of my loft in East Oakland, I welcomed moving to San Francisco in 1995 and found a comfortable space in a safe, residential neighborhood that has been my refuge ever since. Finding a studio became more challenging and continues to be in flux, a constant pressure on my limited resources as an artist.

My community had grown to include a small but active group of Iranian artists, writers, and scholars who produced educational and cultural programming in the Bay Area. I soon became involved with Darvag Theater in Berkeley, a small theater space in a dilapidated building on Ashby Avenue where many members of the Iranian diaspora community gathered regularly. Darvag produced original short plays, creating a platform to share firsthand experiences of exile and survival amidst the political turmoil of the prior decade. Working within this vibrant creative community of makers has continued to fuel my soul. Many collaborations and partnerships have sprouted through the years in a number of projects. An awarded residency at The Lab and funding from New Langton Arts allowed me to envision creating spaces for conversations and platforms for creative exchange within and across my two communities, a continuous focus in my work in the following decades. We came together for conversations, creative actions, and storytelling that culminated in performances with Darvag. Gathered wishes, memories, and stories of women were embedded in the structures and became the soundscape of the space at The Lab (*Sacred Space*, 1995).

My husband, Mohsen Emaminouri, was a newcomer to the U.S. after years of living in Vienna, Austria, when we met through a family connection in 1997. He is another Iranian dreamer of my generation, committed to fighting for a just society and striving for social change. Creating a home together in the Bay Area has allowed me to feel more grounded and gradually experience the lifting of a sustained anxiety and loss that for decades had been ingrained in my displaced body. Energized by our partnership, and with his support, I took on several ambitious community projects in 2000 that anchored my role as an organizer and curator and defined my path as an artist. Creating archives of collected stories, wishes, images, and memories of my diaspora communities became a quest: to save, to savor, to share, and to create understanding. These archives created opportunities for creative exchange with artists, writers, and scholars that revealed our multidimensional, layered stories and diverse expressions, taking control of our own narrative.

I became a U.S. citizen in 2000. The Iranian community in the diaspora was growing roots and the relationship between Iran and the United States seemed on the mend. The purchase of a building in Berkeley by the Persian Center, an Iranian cultural organization, inspired me to propose a project that would bring the community together to share their stories and reflect their images and narratives within the mirrored walls of its gathering hall for generations to come. We proposed and were awarded a Creative Work Fund grant for the *Hall of Reflections* project. The project allowed us to create connections across generations of Iranian communities dispersed around Northern California and offered a much-needed space for dialogue about the rapid changes we were experiencing as Iranian immigrants in the political climate of post-9/11 America. *Hall of Reflections* was also awarded a San Francisco Arts Commission Cultural Equity grant as well as a Story Fund from California Humanities. Fueling the project, however, was the support of many community members who shared their stories and gave wholeheartedly with their time and resources. We produced over 400 glass and mirror assemblages that came together brick by brick to build endless configurations and patterns.

The tiles from the *Hall of Reflections* were installed in the San Francisco Arts Commission Gallery in fall 2002. It went on to exhibit at the Sharjah International Biennial 6, curated by Hoor Al Qasimi and Peter Lewis, in March 2003, coinciding with the start of the bombing of Baghdad by America. The installation was transformed, becoming an echo of the destruction and the displacement of millions that we were witnessing daily. It was a perplexing time being so close to the center of the conflict while engaging in conversations with the many refugees of the unending wars. It was also inspiring to connect to so many international artists, including a few from the emerging Iranian art scene that was attracting global attention. These relationships have grown through the years, creating connections to a global community of artists whose diasporic experiences, shared history, mythology, rituals, and poetry are woven through their works, which are affected deeply by the politics of our times.

Trying to make sense of the complexity of the histories that has shaped the path of my life has led to collecting and archiving projects that invite conversations across diverse communities. CrossConnections (2005–06), an artist residency project at the Center for Art and Public Life (CAPL) at California College of the Arts (CCA), invited an intergenerational Bay Area group of writers, artists, and performers of Iranian heritage to gather regularly over a year to reflect on their shared, layered, and diverse experiences. Dr. Sonia BasSheva Mañjon, the center's director, was instrumental in creating the opportunity for me to offer several courses as part of my residency which ignited my passion for teaching that has continued to this day; teaching when time allowed, and more recently as ranked faculty at CCA. We, along with my scholar-collaborator Dr. Persis Karim, applied for The Christensen Fund grant that focused on stories of the diaspora communities in the Bay Area. Their funding made possible a year of programming, workshops, and exhibitions. Working closely with Kevin Chen, artistic director at the Intersection for the Arts, we took over the two-story building for two weeks, creating temporary murals that filled two flights of stairs with selected phrases drawn from our collective dialogues. This led to an immersive hundred-year historical timeline documented through news headlines, with participants' creative responses to selected dates (*Of Past and Present*, 2005). The project was expanded with performances at Oliver Center Gallery in RePresent exhibition at CCA later that summer.

The exhibition at Intersection for the Arts was the beginning of a series of collaborations with Kevin Chen, first with a solo exhibition *Most Wanted* (2007) which offered the opportunity for me to create several ambitious, site-responsive works in response to rising Islamophobia in this country. I was also offered their theater space to organize film screenings, poetry readings, and performances. Kevin and I continued working together on the exhibition *One Day, a Collective Narrative of Tehran* (2009), inviting participation of a number of contemporary artists living in Iran with the help of artist Ghazaleh Hedayat who had returned back to Iran after her studies at the San Francisco Art Institute.

For over two decades I have been motivated to create safe spaces of gathering and creative exchange, often around challenging, uncomfortable truths, many of which have taken the shape of collective projects, exhibitions, installations, performances, and public art projects. At times, the projects have taken over my studio practice and required an exorbitant number of resources and collaborations. However, they have also allowed me to engage with brilliant artists from across the diaspora of Iranian communities living in Iran, Europe, Canada, and across the United States. Funding from Creative Capital (2012), the Center for Innovation in the Arts, Fleishhacker Foundation, Zellerbach Foundation, California Humanities, and other direct support of my projects has allowed me to continue to work independently with institutions and galleries to launch exhibitions, programming, and workshops contributing to creating a sense of a growing artist community in the Bay Area. This includes a large survey exhibition entitled *Once at Present* at the Minnesota Street Project in 2019, featuring the emerging voices of Bay Area Iranian artists, funded by The Center for Iranian Diaspora Studies at San Francisco State University.

The support of curator Rose Issa, who was among the first to bring the works of artists of the region to the attention of the Western artworld, was crucial to broadening my audience through several exhibitions and publications she produced across Europe and the Middle East until the closing of her London gallery in 2019. I have also benefited greatly from the support of numerous independent curators as well as Bay Area non-profit art organizations along the way with commissions, exhibitions, residencies, and awards including Southern Exposure, Kala Art Institute, Montalvo Arts Center, San Francisco Arts Education Project, Luggage Store, California Institute of Integral Studies, and Yerba Buena Center for the Arts. Artsource Consulting provided a great opportunity to create my first permanent public art project (*Ever Green*, 2022) which opened possibilities of explorations in creating large-scale, site-specific public artwork that are often inspired to provide a platform for gathering and contemplation.

At several points on this long journey, I have questioned my path and every time I have come to renew my commitment to continue to create against all odds, even if it meant giving up a more comfortable life, or any kind of social or family life. Financial limitations have affected every aspect of my life and art-making throughout. Income generated from teaching, commissions, sales, public art projects, exhibitions, and occasional curations have continued to be the patchwork of resources that have allowed for the continuation of my practice.

I am at times critical of the blinding passion that was planted in my heart so early on that has in one way or another directed every decision in my life, but I have never known a different reality. My passion for creating has also saved me many times, giving me a tool for expression through very difficult years, while witnessing so many of my peers perishing. Ultimately, I am grateful to have had the chance to be able to devote some of my life to making, sharing, and developing an ability to communicate with the language of the senses that has connected me with others. I have also been blessed with working with so many brilliant artists and curators through the years, and it is gratifying to see a growing and vibrant multi-generational community of Iranian artists with flourishing careers active in the Bay Area.

Still here, still committed to my work, to do what I can to create connections across cultures and communities, collaborating and creating opportunities for others when possible, I continue to create projects focused on social change and to be of service to my many communities. At the same time, organizing, teaching, learning, and volunteer work continue to fill a large portion of my time, while I continue to explore new paths in the creation and presentation of my work. •

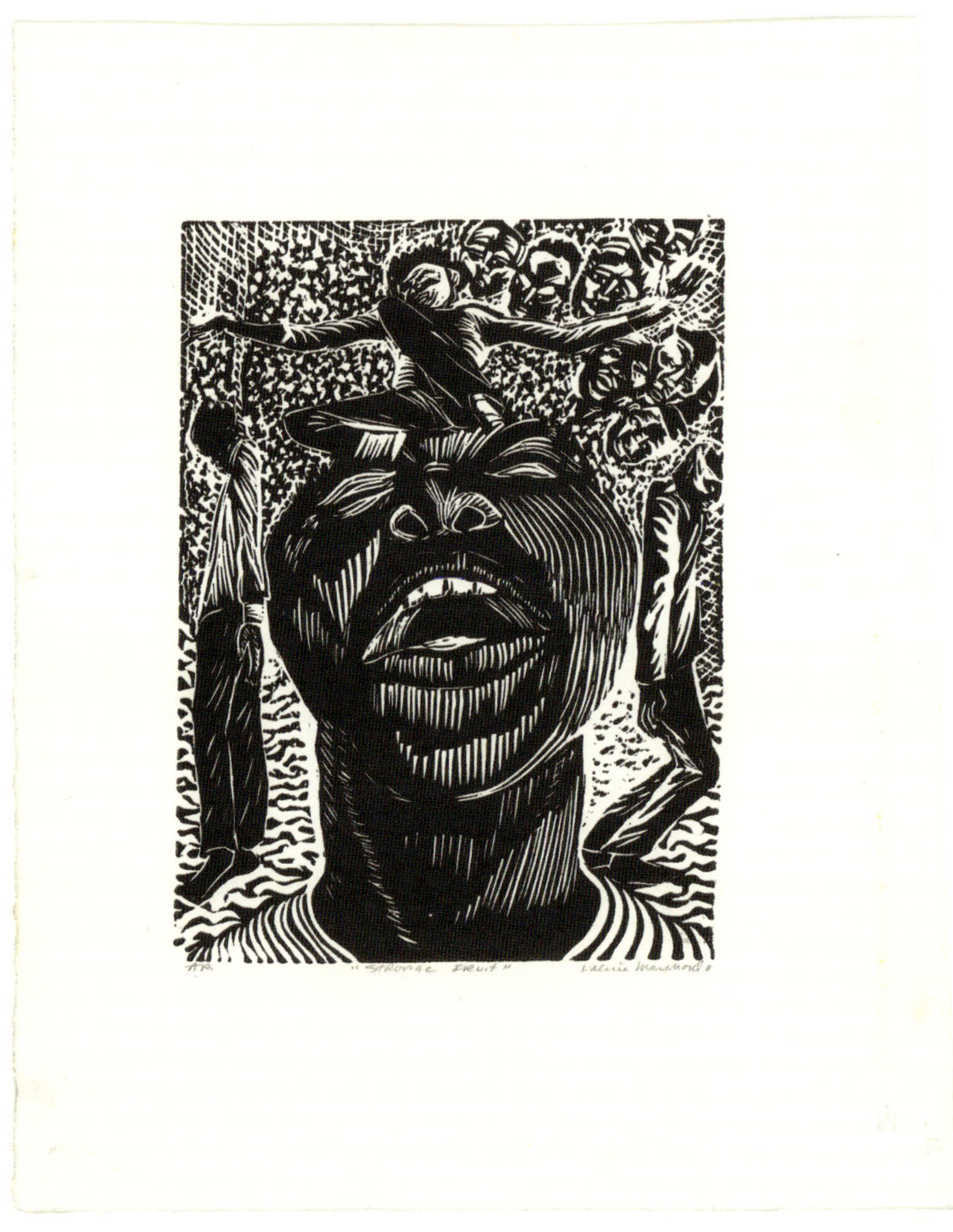
A.P.
"Strange Fruit"
Valerie Maynard

I WAS BORN IN Harlem at the Harlem Hospital and lived right across from the Schomburg Library. Every parade came through my block, and I am thinking as a kid that the parade was coming through everybody's block, but it came through my block because the armory, river, and everything ended there. This is Harlem. Things have changed. My grandparents lived a block over on Lennox Ave, between 7th and 8th. I grew up attending Adam Clayton Powell's church, Abyssinian Baptist Church, so that brought on another kind of consciousness because he was always talking about what we needed to do. People came from all over the world to attend that church. It wasn't just "amen," and "thank you ma'am." In those days my father was a bartender, so I watched people talking about their experiences with him. You saw everybody. It fostered my political understanding of the world. Everything was going on without it being compartmentalized. It affected me, I wasn't aware of how unique that was, to be in that time right there in that place with the Daughters of Ruth and Masons and organizers who were picketing in the streets because they couldn't find jobs. People on soap boxes. Every kind of person, religion, belief was all in my neighborhood. Some of my early drawings as a teenager would be of those people; someone playing checkers on the sidewalk or people talking.

I was an apprentice of a French portrait painter Elaine Journey in New Rochelle. She would be there in the daytime and I had

Valerie Maynard
*Strange Fruit*
1960
12 1/2″x10 1/2″
Woodcut

Courtesy of The Valerie J. Maynard Foundation and the New York Public Library the night and weekends. I don't remember what I wrote to apply, but she said that she didn't call anybody but me. It was great to finally have a space, and they had money and threw away stuff, so I had access to paints and pencils. Elaine was a cellist as well as a portrait painter, and her father was the designer for Paris operas, so she grew up sitting in the seats drawing people on the stage. She would travel during the summer to Tanglewood. The whole summer I could use the space. That is the first real space that I had that I could use to make art. I used to bike up there, from Harlem to New Rochelle, so my father bought me my first scooter.

After that I worked several odd jobs; the telephone company, the post office, Macy's. I had places I would sit all over the boroughs and just watch and draw. I did that all over the city. We were raised to swim, bike, and ice skate, so I did all that stuff. We would never spend a nickel on the bus or the train, we would walk. We walked everywhere. From Harlem to Brooklyn or anywhere. It was safe to do then. I was very adventurous.

I was a super for a few buildings. Did it on the East Side 7th street, Uptown Broadway, 167th street, so I always had a space in those buildings to work. I would usually get the winos to do the maintenance work for me. I know my way around a boiler and other things too. I've always been savvy with mechanical things. While I was doing that I also worked with community centers and youth, I worked in theaters. I built lofts for awhile. I made shoes and bags. I can make anything until I get bored with it.

I worked at The Sculpture House for a while around 1956–57. I went there to get a job so that I could learn more tools, and that was the place for sculpture in New York. The brothers cast and sold sculpture supplies. I worked behind the counter and made friends with a guy from Puerto Rico who made the tools and I could call him up and describe the tool to him and he would meet me at the train with it. Another sculpture supply couple who lived on 1st or 2nd Avenue down on the East Side, Stanley, and I can't recall his wife's name, and he would call me up and say, "Kiss your sugar daddy and get over here, we got something for you!" They would go to Italy once a year to buy stones and get mallets made. Once a year, they would save all of their money and go. I had a lot of allies who could fix things or offer supplies. I learned a lot from people in hardware stores and mom-and-pop supplies stores.

I started off working on portraits in the 1960s. I stopped doing portraits because those who posed always had critiques like, “don’t paint my right side” or “don’t draw me from that angle.” I drew fast and only charged one dollar a minute. I wasn’t getting any money, so I dropped it. After portraits I was working in the theater and worked for the park department. That was the longest-running job I ever had. I worked the East Side Tompkins Square Park, and Washington Square Park in the West Village, in the summers. All of the poets and writers, what folks called bohemians, would congregate in the plaza of Washington Square Park. I would go to dance studios in Albany. I loved dance and all the theater stuff. I could sew and make shoes, so I started doing those things. I was never serious in it; it didn’t hold me.

I taught myself to print at the Studio Museum of Harlem. There was no print workshop there before my residency, so I created one. I went to Bob Blackburn, who had a shop in Manhattan. I told him that I needed a press and he gave me a contact to get my own press. He was an amazing man, an amazing printmaker. He had a shop for many years, he remembered everyone, your name and the country you were from. I made a few lithographs there and I set up my press in an old dress factory. This was in the 1960s.

I had a loft on 126th St. I started a gallery where I could put work, not my work, in peoples’ offices and it would stay a month or so and then I would switch the work out with new art. A woman had started a Black employment agency in the 1940s and I was switching some work in there when I met a guy who offered me the opportunity to go to Poland Spring, Maine, to work with youth. I agreed and when I arrived I was the only person there from the city who had worked in community centers, camps, or parks. He later offered me a job to do that work full time, so I set up an organization called Arts for Living based on a query about how we could live our lives without putting a dollar down, basically teaching people how to live without debt. Students would learn how to sow, make their own shoes, or anything they needed to live. The program became the largest job corp. in the country.

My brother was arrested in 1970 and I came and found a place, a basement studio in Hunts Point in the Bronx, and I was looking for a lawyer for him. I traveled all over the city trying to find a lawyer. James Wechsler, a reporter on the *NY Post*, began to write things about my brother and his trial, which was a stroke of great luck. I started sculpting around then. I had no money, so I made and sold prints, did trade and barter and held fundraisers to cover legal fees. For the seven years that he was in jail, that is all I did. After 2,177 days my brother was released. By the time he was released I had a studio on 126th street across from Morningside.

When you see artists now, all they do is their art. I was never that person. I grew up in a community and we did everything. In Harlem, you are a part of everything. I never thought about the work I was making as going toward a career as an artist. I did everything. I used to make medallions and social commentary works, quick sketches about what I saw. I loved working for the park department because I had a lot of fun with the kids. I have always been attracted to wilderness and water—both are spiritual places. I participated in many artist residencies including the Blue Mountain Center in New York, The Walker Institute, Brandywine Graphic Workshop, MacDowell Colony, and Massachusetts Institute of Technology (M.I.T.), among others. Residencies are a way of transcending the space you are in—finding fluidity. I met a lot of interesting people. The studio is a sacred space for me. I didn't have the same kind of regiment as other artists who attended the residency. I didn't have the same constraints. I think I have always been an anomaly in those spaces—always moving in my own rhythm.

I have always been an explorer of buildings. They always thought I was the maid, so no one ever stopped me. One day I walked into the Art Students League and spoke with a guard who told me I should meet the director, who shared an opportunity to attend a residency in Vermont. I went there for the summer and worked with Native American and Haitian sculptors. I carved my first stone there. While I was carving a clay head, some of the older sculptors corrected the way I was doing it—they had all gone to school and learned the proper way to sculpt.

The first major public work I completed is on 126th and 3rd avenue at the City of New York Multi-Service Center. I knew the architect of the building in Harlem, Jerry Barr. I was commissioned to make a ceramic bas-relief (11 × 16.5 inches) for his building while in residence at the Studio Museum of Harlem running the print workshop. During that time, the Studio Museum was just a few lofts overtop a liquor store. We knew everybody on the block, every kind of person you could find in Harlem, and they knew us.

I never thought that art-making was all that there is. I was never just an artist. I had to eat. I had to pay rent, but I wasn't making art to do those things. I know that the rest of the world was part of the world too, not just because I was an artist. I felt a responsibility to us, to a community that would not allow me to be just an artist. I knew that I wanted to do public works and do something that wouldn't be painted over. I wanted to do work that wasn't commercial.

Right now I am trying to finish the work that I started. I have many finished and unfinished works. I am an artist, but now my focus is on finishing works, archiving, and mentoring. Some of the so-called students of mine are grandmothers now. I am happy to still be living. Day by day I digest new things. My life as an artist has not been compartmentalized; from the ground up and everyplace I have been or made work in, life has informed my art-making practice. The privilege of being alive, seeing people grow, seeing what the battles are, what the battles will always be, what the love is, everything influences me and has influenced my work. What's really important to me these days is finding some nature, being in the woods and just being there. There, you are connecting to yourself, to your human-being-ness. ●

# CONCLUSION

Raheleh Filsoofi

THERE ARE millions of artists all over the world who inspire, serve, and are depended on in their local communities. Thanks to asking friends from the Ceramic Society in Tehran, I discovered three important women who define what identity, strength, and perseverance mean aside from their age.

Over the course of a few months, I learned how potters lived, how they thought, how they loved, and how they made pottery part of their daily routines.

Ms. Ahdiyeh Roshanfekr at the village of Jirdeh (Central Gillan province), Ms. Fatemeh Mohebi at the village of Khomar Mahaleh (East Gillan), and Ms. Sara Mohamadi at the City of Marand (West Azerbaijan province) are all more than just makers of ceramics. They all have children and extended families. Some of the women have gone through various trauma, such as one of the women who lost her son in a motorcycle accident.

I visited this group of women in 2012 and 2015, and then stayed connected with them until the pandemic began in 2020. The village where I visited in 2012 is located in North Iran, which is known to have strong women and more open spaces for women-makers who came from different backgrounds and have families of their own. While Iran is a country that does not recognize human rights for women, these women have conquered adversity throughout their lives and at the same time, have made ceramics for others to use and enjoy.

The women I visited were of different ages and looked much older than they actually were. I can only guess that was because they took care of others more than themselves, which includes their family, friends, and those in their village. They dressed traditionally, working as they led others to work, engaged in the kitchen, studio, and land. Ms. Roshanfekr, Ms. Mohebi, and Ms. Mohamadi are all vested in making their artwork as a part of their daily lives.

What struck me most was the hidden beauty and sublime power of their simple, abstract presence. These women worked as leaders in their communities, creating art, supporting their families, and providing jobs and opportunities for others. Away from the restrictive rules and regulations of life in Tehran and other major cities, these women constructed a safe space for their families and communities to create work.

Of my still vibrant memories of my visits, one day stands out. After a long conversation with Mrs. Mohebi, I re-entered her studio after everyone else had left. I had a chance to immerse myself in its simple beauty. The work produced there might not be sufficiently sophisticated to the eyes of the Western ceramic world, but the pristine craftsmanship and the purity of the display of the pieces in a dim and humble studio made them remarkable. Their work and their dignity greatly influenced my installations later on: the light, the material, the presentation of their work in their storage rooms, their guilelessness. These are values that rise above any specific technique, style, or subject matter in their creations. Transfixed by such simplicity and honesty, my artistic and intellectual life was forever changed in that storage room. The dispositions and attributes, the essence of artistic practice that had eluded me in the academic world of the West, was realized in the modest and unpretentious studio of a woman potter in a small village in Iran.

You can call these women contemporary artists. But gatekeepers in the contemporary art world may not see them as such. In some ways, they are true contemporary, working artists who serve their communities in many different ways. They don't look at themselves as artists, but rather make ceramics as a way to take care of others; as providers and leaders rather than "artists." What they were doing in their village made them visible and that was enough for them. It showed me that you have to make a difference where you are, in the community in which you live.

Observing their normalities, I was struck as to how confident they were. They knew who they were, where they were, and trusted themselves and others around them. The source of this confidence was from the community they were and are a part of today.

The kinds of ceramics they made varied. One of the women was making a sculpture inspired by others, and the two other women made functional pieces to serve, to make food, to eat and drink from. Whether their work was deemed "artistic" or "useful" had no hierarchical value: all of the objects they made came from the same places of love, dedication to others, and sources of pride. They were also very trusting of the medium they were working with, that the medium was serving all of their purposes. They were making something without expectation, timeless, to be used by others, all aware of the processes in front of them. They held a consistent, strong belief and understanding of their processes, all of which was very clear and mindful.

These women lived a simple life. They didn't have many tools, space, etc. – they were working with whatever they had, whatever the community provided, content with what they had. It taught me that you can work with what is available.

This group of women was so impactful to me, my work, and practice; they were a strong example of artists' importance in society and their local communities. The interactions with them have affected how I live and work in my life. The model by which they serve their community through the practice of building ceramics is a model that is not seen in the contemporary artworld, but in the village.

Ms. Ahdiyeh Roshanfekr, Ms. Fatemeh Mohebi, and Ms. Sara Mohamadi were committed, dedicated to what they were making and not deterred by the opinions of others.

They were persistent in their leadership and powerful in their communities but also in ceramics: the media that they controlled with authority and grace, in making their work. A constant part of their life, at the highest quality that they demanded was met.

There was no shame in selling their work themselves to further engage in their community, a responsibility they owned. Their presence and consistency in making and presenting had everything to do with them being women and their power. They were examples of courage in a country that was at odds with them. They believed in what they did and still do today.

Where they are practicing is very different from where contemporary art is shown in Tehran. They are protected by their villages. They have complete freedom in their communities because they are part of the thread by which the community lives.

I was born in Tehran, in the midst of a revolution. As I grew into adulthood, after the revolution and the war, I became increasingly aware of, and affected by, the limitations imposed on women. I chose to seek my future elsewhere, where I felt there would be more opportunity and less restrictions, where I thought I would not have to clamber up the slope constantly struggling against adversity.

Traditions continue because mentorship is carried through from mentors' lives to others. This continues due to their strength, having forged paths for others. I am proud to share their stories, as a catalyst to show paths that they have built for me and others. Never to die, beyond their living on this earth. Their resiliency is within me every day, and I continue to share their practices and models of living with what I teach, how I work in the studio, and how I interact with those in my community.

"The work" that will last for a lifetime are memories of the women themselves, because all of their commitment to their community was centered on the ceramics they made, but incredibly so much more. The work brings people together. They are *the glue* and backbone to the community in engagement, experiences, growth, love, and memories of one another. The ceramics are the center of so much. The object becomes a manifestation of their existence, connection, presence, and more.

A constant reminder of the truth and certainty that supports and motivates me is the strong presence of women in this most recent protest. The slogan of "Women, Life, Freedom" is an indication of their fearless determination. The new generation of Iranian women was raised by the generations of Iranian women who have tried to claim their space and find their own voice in society despite the challenges. I can only hope they will succeed where others have not. I will not relent. I will not be deterred. I will push this rock to the top of the mountain. I will persevere for my efforts to be heard, to be seen, to be acknowledged for them, for me, for us.

Ms. Ahdiyeh Roshanfekr, Ms. Fatemeh Mohebi, and Ms. Sara Mohamadi and their practices opened doors to me, helped me understand and re-evaluate the notion of my own identity as an Iranian woman and more importantly as an artist. While people take pride in celebrating artists showing on white walls, separated in an exclusive world that does not recognize artists such as these women, my duty as a witness is to share their stories, their model of a working artist today, and how important artists are to their communities. ●

# CONCLUSION

Shervone Neckles

FOR TEN YEARS, I served as the artist programs manager of professional development at the Joan Mitchell Foundation and co-editor of *Creating A Living Legacy (CALL): Career Documentation for Visual Artists. CALL* is an initiative designed to assist artists in shaping their legacy by positioning themselves, their work, and their critical concerns within art history. Throughout this period, I have actively engaged in extensive conversations focusing on the various ways to ensure artists are duly acknowledged and remembered for their invaluable contributions to society. This role has afforded me the privilege of collaborating with and learning from an esteemed group of visual artists, as well as art, business, and legal professionals from across the United States.

From 2013 to 2023, I collaborated with 27 *CALL* artists and assisted four national partner organizations in adapting their own *CALL* program model, collectively supporting thirty visual artists. To fully understand the significance of an artist taking ownership of the documentation and preservation of their life's work and personal legacy, I collaborated with a diverse spectrum of visual artists, ranging in ages from their mid-50s to early 90s. It was crucial that the fieldwork was inclusive to the diverse needs of the artists. I worked closely with artists with a variety of abilities, cultural backgrounds, geographical locations, professional practices, personal values, intentions, career points, and financial circumstances.

The participating artists were all contending with common barriers in the legacy-planning process. Each faced the challenges of entering the documentation process at a later stage in their careers. Each maintained prolific, multifaceted studio practices with substantial volumes of artwork and records that required a more efficient organization and inventorying systems, enabling them to leverage career-advancing opportunities. Unlike more resourced studios with fully operational teams and gallery administration support to assist in the day-to-day business, production, and access to next-level professional networks and opportunities, these artists were at the early stages of implementing their strategic planning resources, identifying suitable tools and tailoring the technology to meet their specific needs. These were essential elements for developing a long-term vision for their artistic legacies, inevitably empowering them to create a comprehensive career documentation and inventory management system. Their ongoing endeavor is to sustain their artistic vision by assembling a support team of trusted, knowledgeable, qualified individuals who believe in their vision and are invested in helping them connect their artwork and archive to future generations.

Every interaction with an artist on this journey has expanded my view of what it means to live one's values and pursue a lifelong artistic practice. These artists persist and continue to make their work regardless of obstacles, always maintaining hope and determination. I am humbled by the countless selfless gestures and acts of generosity I have witnessed firsthand between artists, the communities they live and work in, and even the industry they help to thrive. For example, one artist I worked with prioritized community needs by establishing a non-profit social justice art organization in the late 1960s. Operational to this day, it serves children, creates job opportunities for artists, and provides quality art education experiences for students from elementary to college-level and adults.

In another example, an artist leverages personal connections to support fellow artists within their community challenged by systemic oppression. They created a platform that intentionally fostered connections between trusted scholars, art professionals, the next generation of artists, and elders. This platform presents exhibitions, artist interviews, and other texts aimed at documenting and preserving the significant contributions of their community to society.

My undergraduate and graduate education never covered the many lessons I received from these artists, such as their origin stories, managing family ties, charting a career path, building an inner circle of support, handling fluctuating relationships with money, and navigating the gallery and museum systems. There is so much untapped potential for the artworld to gain insights and learn from the rich history and lives of these pioneering artists and their archives. Their artwork and records serve as tangible evidence of their human activity, observations, and civic engagement. It is an incredible loss to the field, and a true disservice to future generations, when we fail to fully recognize their impact and fail to credit their influential work in fueling the contemporary art discourse of today.

Just as higher education needs amending, so do the ways in which contemporary artists work with gallery dealers. For instance, an artist, while organizing their inventory and records, reached out to their gallery for information only to discover that the gallery was in total disarray. Because of the gallery's lack of organization, the artist missed out on opportunities. Consequently, the artist assumed control of managing their work and career and severed ties with that gallery so they could forge new relationships. Despite the immediate heartbreak and disruption caused by the discovery, the experience fundamentally shifted the way the artist manages their studio and their expectations and reliance on galleries going forward.

These seasoned artists possess a profound understanding of knowledge production that significantly contributes to the brilliance of their work. Their unwavering conviction and sense of purpose propel them beyond fear, rejection, and even the possibility of never being recognized. Spending time with them, immersing myself in their presence, sharing their spaces, and engaging them in conversations about the evolution of their work have profoundly impacted me, and I believe it has the potential to do the same for others. Just being in proximity with them injected surges of adrenaline into my creative process, providing fuel for weeks of heightened productivity. Reflecting intimately with these artists spurred my own personal growth, helping me define my role as an artist and how I can be of service to a larger purpose. This purpose is reflected in my own work, which preserves memories and histories, as well as in my advocacy work with fellow artists. If these encounters with seasoned artists can have a transformative effect on me, imagine the possibilities if more opportunities existed for intergenerational groups of artists to engage and collaborate—not just for work or mentorship, but for genuine friendship.

I am profoundly grateful for the artists who, with their wealth of knowledge gained from a lifetime of experiences, have left an indelible mark. The stories and struggles of these artists provided me with affirmation, reinforcing the significance of my own voice and work. Seeing myself as part of a continuum, I recognize that, along with my peers, it is our responsibility to contribute back and foster collective strength in our community. There is no way to convey the amount of respect and acknowledgement due to the generations that precede me. However, as a witness to these dedicated artists who labored and paved the way for myself and my fellow artists, I consider it my duty to carry their legacy forward in my lifelong commitment as an artist to myself, my practice, and my community. •

# ACKNOWLEDGMENTS

PUTTING THIS book together was a slow process that demanded patience through the starts and stops and endless delays due to the pandemic and other personal issues. I certainly could not have produced it without the tremendous assistance, feedback, mentorship, generosity, kindness, and referrals from the many who believed in this project.

The artist contributors who gave their histories for all of us to learn from are to be admired. It is with the utmost respect that I express my gratitude to them for their time, efforts, and, certainly, their incredible stories. Their journeys are beacons of light for all of us to follow.

Thank you to the Valerie J. Maynard Foundation for their assistance and permission to publish Valerie's essay for this book. Valerie was gracious, strong, and such an amazing mentor to many. Even though Valerie passed away in September 2022, the power of her voice will always resonate through her work and writing.

In addition, I am extremely grateful to Katinka Mann's children for their enthusiastic efforts and response in the publishing of her mother's important essay. Katinka was such a joyful, beautiful person, and although deeply saddened at her passing in August 2022, I am comforted by hearing her voice through her words in this book. Her light-hearted spirit continues to shine brightly through her essay.

After this manuscript was completed, Audrey Flack suddenly passed away in June 2024. Audrey was (and remains) dear to my heart, as she was a fierce, courageous woman unafraid to share her opinions. Her voice is vividly present and alive in this essay; I can still hear it as clearly as if it were yesterday. While writing this essay, she was also working on her memoir, *With Darkness Came Stars: A Memoir*. I miss her terribly.

The process of narrowing down what Audrey would share in her essay was guided with the assistance of Severin Delfs, who was then Audrey Flack's Studio Manager. I am deeply grateful to Severin for our conversations and for his collaboration with Audrey, which made it possible for her essay to appear here.

Thank you to the Two Old Bitches (Idelisse Malavé and Joanne Sanders), Raheleh Filsoofi, and Shervone Neckles for their strong bookends to the essays. Your perspectives are comforting and validating to many artists who are persevering with their artistic practices in the later years of their lives.

To all the photographers who generously contributed images of the artists' works that were selected for this book, we appreciate your contribution. Photographs of the artwork accompanying each essay were essential.

Special recognition goes to my wonderful friends who directed me to some of the contributors in this book, including Valerie Cassel Oliver, Shervone Neckles, Alpesh Kantilal Patel, Mark Tribe, Houry Geudelekian, Namita Gupta Wiggers, Austin Thomas, Leslie Gerber-Seid, and Hrag Vartanian. Thank you for your thoughtful suggestions and the great work you do everyday in amplifying the voices of artists all over the world.

Darren Walker has changed my life in many ways. I am deeply grateful to him—not only for who he is, but for the pathways he has built for me and others, and for the countless lives he has uplifted. Without his belief in me, along with the support of the Ford Foundation, the conversation tour for our previous two books would not have been possible. Darren continues to inspire me with his strength as a true change-maker, and for his generosity, I am profoundly thankful.

A big thanks goes to Ruby Lerner, who has taught me so much about advocacy and leadership. Her mentorship continues to fuel the work I do. I continue to learn from her by way of her archives and just being in her space: Ruby being Ruby—a treasure who is also a strong force in the world.

Going back even further, I must acknowledge the important role that my high school art teacher, Mary Bloom, gifted me as the first person in my life to show me the pathway toward a life as an artist.

To Amy Damutz, who first approached me in 2011 to submit a proposal to Intellect Books, and the entire team of exceptional people there in Bristol, UK: I am so grateful for our great work together. The work we do together remains meaningful, timely and important. Thank you for your continued commitment to making a place for artists' journeys to be told.

To those who continue to support my overall work as an artist, especially fellow-advocates for artists, I am thankful you have included me in your community without judgement or prejudice. You are an integral part of the success of this book and all I do.

Thank you to the more than 350 artists who applied to my open call to be considered for inclusion in this book. While the timing wasn't right for me to include your story, it was nonetheless inspiring to read your histories, all of which have contributed to my research of our vibrant community.

The Living and Sustaining a Creative Life series of books remain a powerful foundation for conversation, which has led to real, pragmatic pathways and solutions for artists to continue to live their creative lives. My first and second book tours would not have happened without donors to our Kickstarter fundraiser more than ten years ago. Nor would all 164 stops have been possible without the contributors to our ongoing fiscally-sponsored book tour project. Combined with the foundations who generously supported both tours, we were able to cross-pollinate and connect many of those 80 contributors with nearly 10,000 other creative minds in different communities throughout the United States and abroad. These artist-to-artist conversations highlighted how we are just hardworking people like any other profession. Yet they also reinforced how artists play important and essential roles in our society, validating our entire series of books that are focusing on other disciplines in forthcoming publications. Without the support of all these donors, we would not have been able to forge important, meaningful partnerships over the years. Thank you!

Finally, my deepest gratitude goes to the love of my life, Vinson Valega, my partner in everything I do. His participation in this book was crucial in every aspect. Our journey is evergreen. •